THE/CUT

Lose Up to 10 Pounds in 10 Days
and Sculpt Your Best Body

**Morris Chestnut and
Obi Obadike, MS, CFT, SFN**

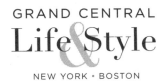

GRAND CENTRAL
Life & Style
NEW YORK · BOSTON

Copyright © 2017 by Morris Chestnut and Obi Obadike

Cover design by Lisa Honerkamp. Cover photography by Noel Daganta.
Cover copyright © 2017 by Hachette Book Group, Inc.

Grand Central Life & Style
Hachette Book Group
1290 Avenue of the Americas
New York, NY 10104
grandcentrallifeandstyle.com
twitter.com/grandcentralpub

First Edition: April 2017

Grand Central Life & Style is an imprint of Grand Central Publishing.
The Grand Central Life & Style name and logo are trademarks of Hachette Book Group, Inc.

The publisher is not responsible for websites (or their content) that are not owned by the publisher.

The Hachette Speakers Bureau provides a wide range of authors for speaking events. To find out more, go to www.hachettespeakersbureau.com or call (866) 376-6591.

Exercise photos by Noel Daganta.

Library of Congress Cataloging-in-Publication Data
Names: Chestnut, Morris, author. | Obadike, Obi, author.
Title: The cut : lose up to 10 pounds in 10 days and sculpt your best body / Morris Chestnut and Obi Obadike.
Description: First edition. | Boston : Grand Central Life & Style, [2017] | Includes bibliographical references and index.
Identifiers: LCCN 2016029301| ISBN 9781455565238 (hardback) | ISBN 9781478970033 (audio download) | ISBN 9781455565221 (e-book)
Subjects: LCSH: Weight loss—Popular works. | Reducing exercises—Popular works. | BISAC: HEALTH & FITNESS / Diets. | HEALTH & FITNESS / Weight Loss. | HEALTH & FITNESS / Exercise.
Classification: LCC RM222.2 .C476 2017 | DDC 613.7/12—dc23 LC record available at https://lccn.loc.gov/2016029301

ISBNs: 978-1-4555-6523-8 (hardcover), 978-1-4555-6522-1 (ebook)

Printed in the United States of America

LSC-C

10 9 8 7 6 5 4 3 2 1

From Morris:

I'd like to dedicate this book to all of those who have the courage to take control of their lives. It's an extremely daunting and challenging endeavor but unbelievably rewarding and fulfilling. Good luck!

From Obi:

To Gayle Tucker, who passed away from pancreatic cancer on April 10, 2016. RIP Gayle; you will be greatly missed.

Contents

Part Four: Think to Get Cut

Acknowledgments

From Morris:

I'd first like to thank God for giving me the courage and ability to endure life and its tremendous challenges.

I'd like to acknowledge my parents, Morris and Shirley Chestnut, for raising me with confidence, humility, grace, and class.

I'd like to acknowledge my sister, Carmen, and brother, Mark, for their encouragement and contributions to my childhood.

I'd like to acknowledge my wife, Pamela, and children, Grant and Paige, for their unwavering support and belief in me. They are truly my daily inspiration.

I'd also like to thank my coauthor and great friend Obi Obadike. This book wouldn't have happened if it weren't for him—his vision made this happen. I appreciate our partnership and most importantly, your friendship.

Thanks to Katherine Latshaw, of Folio Literary Management, for creating and consummating great opportunities.

Thanks to Kelly James-Enger for her hard work and dedication.

Thanks to Sarah Pelz and our publisher for giving us this tremendous opportunity.

Special thanks for my manager, Brian Wilkins, of LINK Entertainment. Brian, this is another step along our entertainment journey. Many more to come.

From Obi:

Two authors, by themselves, don't make a book happen! I have so many people to thank and acknowledge. I first want to thank and recognize my coauthor, Morris Chestnut, for agreeing to do this book with me. His belief in the Cut program and in our book concept was instrumental in making this book happen, and his influence and star power play key roles in making this book a success! So thanks, Mo, for being the great guy and, most important, great friend that you are!

I want to acknowledge Katherine Latshaw, our literary agent, who worked very hard from editing the book proposal to seeing the book published. You were amazing, Katherine, and I really appreciate you.

I want to give major props to Kelly James-Enger for her advice, support, and all of the countless hours of editing, restructuring, and reformatting for this book. You were an invaluable asset to making this book powerful and strong. Thank you to Leslie Bilderback for the delicious recipes she created for The Cut. I also want to acknowledge Sarah Pelz, our editor, for her belief in our concept and her invaluable input to make sure that this book is successful.

Special thanks to our publisher, especially the marketing team, for making sure everyone knows about the book. I want to also acknowledge Brian Wilkins and Ryan Bundra from LINK Entertainment for believing in this concept and for connecting me with Morris!

I also want to acknowledge the real people who tried The Cut and shared their "Making the Cut" transformation stories for the book. Your success on this program will make every person who reads the book believe that they can attain the same results. Thanks to all of you for your hard work: Oluwole Awosika, Olivia Rose Bolton, Will Capello, Sharad Cara, Renee Carter, William Scott Carter, Osborn H. "Tiger" Christon Jr., Dionne Davis, Rome Douglas, Donna Eggleston, Stacy Ezel, Tyrone Foster, Mike Hopper, Tiaja Pierre, Joey Ray, Jeffrey Smith, and Stevland Turner.

I want to acknowledge my social media team, who does so many amazing things for my brand; thank you Jen Faustner and Herbert Smelik!

I want to thank my entire family and my friends, specifically my mom, dad, and brother, who have consistently supported me.

I also want to thank Bill Phillips, author of *Body for Life*. Without his book's success, *The Cut* might not exist. The transformation concept associated with *Body for Life* planted the seed for the concept behind *The Cut*. So, thank you, Bill, for the inspiration—and for being a great mentor and good friend.

I want to thank Faith For Today, the producers of the *Lifestyle Magazine* show, and the people associated with it, including: Mike Tucker, Gayle Tucker (RIP), Monique Roy, Chauncey Smith, Dr. Sharmini Long, Lynell LaMountain, Jennifer LaMountain,

Jeff Wood, and everybody who is associated with making *Lifestyle Magazine* a successful health television show.

I also want to acknowledge Kelechi Opara and Dr. Jill Kristine Huseman for the support over the last couple of years. You are both beautiful people inside and out. Thanks for always having my back.

Finally, I want to thank all of my fans who have supported me from day one in my fitness career. My goal, ultimately, is to make the world a healthier place, and I hope this book will do so for everyone!

Introduction

It was a winter night in 2012 in New York, where I was staying while shooting a guest appearance on *Nurse Jackie*. I was standing at the window, looking down at the Big Apple, which bustled with life even at 10 minutes before midnight.

The phone rang.

It was director Malcolm Lee with news that *The Best Man Holiday* had just been green-lit. That meant the movie was a go. Great news! Right? It should have been, except I could guess what he was going to want from my character, Lance Sullivan, this time around.

"Morris, I need you to be ripped!"

I agreed to take the part, and hung up the phone. Then anxiety set in. Reality check. At about 220 pounds, I wasn't exactly ripped. In fact, I couldn't see my abs. They were hiding somewhere beneath a layer of fat. I may have looked fine with clothes on, but now I was going to be shot without my shirt on. I'd shot the original *Best Man* movie 13 years before, when I was in my early 30s and a good 30 pounds lighter. Now I wanted to make a statement that even in my 40s, I could be as fit as I was then. The question was, how?

I had only 12 weeks before the show started shooting. How was I going to lose that much weight in that time—especially at my age? I knew I was going to have to work twice as hard as I would have had to in my 20s or even 30s to look the way the director wanted me to. In an industry that is age-conscious, I couldn't afford to appear in front of millions of people—and be captured on film forever—in the kind of shape I was in. It would make a difference in my being able to work as a leading man.

I knew I'd put on some weight, but my current role hadn't required me to take my shirt off on camera. I'd been shooting in New York that December, and skipping workouts. I've also always had a sweet tooth, and I'd been having dessert after nearly every meal. Once I started down that path, the pounds quickly added up.

But now it was time to take action.

I decided I needed a trainer. A friend of mine recommended Obi, and when I saw photos of him, I was impressed. He was ripped! It's easy for a 20-year-old trainer to be ripped, but Obi was in his late 30s, so I knew he was doing something right.

Working with Obi, I shed the weight, and fast. In 12 weeks, I went from 220 pounds to 187. I was surprised at how quickly the pounds and extra flab seemed to just melt away. But I'm going to be real with you: This was difficult. Probably one of the hardest things I've ever had to do.

Yes, the workouts were hard, but the mental switch was even tougher. I was so out of shape when we started working together that it was tough to stay motivated in the beginning, especially before I could really see results. I worked my butt off to get my 44-year-old body in shape. Yeah, I had a few bad days where I didn't follow the diet perfectly. But I didn't quit. And it paid off.

Audiences apparently enjoyed my new look. *The Best Man Holiday* was a box-office smash, and it seemed like all anybody wanted to talk about was my shirtless scenes in the movie. Whenever I went on air to promote it—from *Wendy Williams* to *Dr. Oz* to the *Today* show to *The Talk*—the same clips of my body were played over and over. Instead of asking about my role in the movie, people asked me how I got in such good shape. Obi and I both were bombarded with emails and calls from around the world, all from people wondering the same things: What exercises do you do? What do you eat? *What can I do to get into shape?* In fact, more than two years later, people *still* want to know what I did to look the way I did on screen.

With so many people asking for our secrets, we realized it was time to share them. That's what this book is about! We're finally sharing the program behind my radical transformation—the plan that will help you create your own wonderful before-and-after success story.

Between shooting my show *Rosewood* and promoting movies like *The Perfect Guy*, I'm busier than ever before. But I've kept the body Obi helped me build—a body that I thought I could never get back. He and I decided to write this book to help all the people out there like me—fed up with the way you look and ready to make a change.

I've been there—I know what it feels like to be frustrated with the way you look, and concerned about changing it. I also know how great it feels to have that confidence back when you've done the work and have the results to show for it.

Obi and I aren't into sugarcoating things, so we won't promise you an easy fix. But if you give us 12 weeks, we'll give you the blueprint to help you get your body back—or get an even better body than you've ever had before! We worked together to create a book that would work for anyone who's ready to say "enough!" and get after it.

So let's get going! You've got nothing to lose (but pounds on the scale), and everything to gain.

—Morris Chestnut, February 2016

I had no idea when Morris reached out to me in December 2012 that it was the beginning of not only a friendship, but a book! Morris saw me on the cover of a magazine, posing with a mutual friend. "I've got to get on this guy's program," he told her. When she told him I was a trainer—a body transformation specialist—he looked up my website and was impressed with the client success stories.

Morris and I started out as trainer/client but we quickly became good friends. The same month *The Best Man Holiday* opened, Morris appeared on the cover of *Muscle & Performance*. The hosts of every talk show (*The View*, *The Talk*, *Dr. Oz*, you name it!) showed that cover and peppered him with questions about how he'd gotten in such fantastic shape. After his promotion tour, we were both bombarded with emails, tweets, and Facebook posts about how people could get the same results that Morris did.

We realized we had a plan that worked, and a plan to share with everyone willing to work hard to get in the best shape of their lives. That's the basis of this book, and what we're excited to share with you!

—Obi Obadike, February 2016

Part One

Why The Cut Works

In part one, the first three chapters of this book, you'll learn why it can seem so difficult to lose weight and keep it off. But we only want to make you aware of the challenges before we show you how to overcome them. In this section, you'll also learn about the basic elements of The Cut. We designed it to help *anyone*, of any age, shed body fat and keep it off—for good. In the "Making the Cut" stories you'll meet many real-life people just like you who followed The Cut and lost staggering amounts of weight in just 12 weeks. And in chapter 2, we'll debunk common fitness, nutrition, and weight loss myths—and educate you about the only way to keep your body lean for life.

1 Getting Cut

How to Lose Your Body Fat and Get Your Best Body Ever

"Man! How did you get so lean?"

"How do I get abs like that?"

"Tell me how I can get ripped like you."

"What do I eat to look like you do?"

"You're in your 40s? No way!"

These are the kinds of statements we hear on a daily basis. When you look like you're in shape, people notice. They usually want to know more about how we got this way—and how we stay this way!

Both of us are in the public eye. Because we're recognizable, you'd be surprised at how many men and women hit us up at the gym, on set, at the grocery store, even in public restrooms with all kinds of questions about dieting, losing weight, exercising, you name it...It seems like everyone wants to know what our secret is.

That's why we decided to write this book. We know that with the right diet and exercise plan, you can radically change your body—in just 12 weeks. If you've put on weight over the years, that means getting your old body back. If you've never felt good about how you look, that means building a better body than you've ever had before!

Maybe you're already working out, but you want to get the kind of body that people notice—the kind of body that inspires them to ask you for *your* secret! Maybe you've tried to lose weight or get in shape before, and failed. If that's you, you're not alone. Don't beat yourself up and don't feel discouraged. You probably fell for an unrealistic program or a fad that had no basis in science. Our plan is based on the latest research and scientific studies, coupled with our experience about what kind of diet and exercise plan produces the most dramatic results. That's The Cut. And it works.

Is it really that simple? Well, yeah. That doesn't mean it's easy. We're not going to coddle you. As a pair of alpha males, that's not our style! You've got to have the discipline to follow the program. There's no such thing as a magic pill or shortcut that will give you results.

Our attitude is that if you say you're ready, then you're ready all the way—no BS. If that's you, and you're ready to do the work, we'll give you the blueprint to follow. Your job is to put in the time and the effort and follow that blueprint.

From Obi:

Tired of diet plans not working for you? That's a big reason clients hire me—because I know how to help people get results. As a body transformation specialist, it's my job to help you reach your genetic potential.

I've worked with thousands of people—ranging from Hollywood actors and celebrities to everyday people just like you—to help them lose weight and keep it off. My clients have included all body types, including those who have never been able to change their bodies before. When they put in the work, and follow my plan, they get results.

I promise if you give me 12 weeks of your life, you'll emerge a leaner, stronger, all-around more confident version of you. That's the power of The Cut—and my promise to you.

You'll see real-life examples in this book, and if you want to see more, check out TheCutBook.com.

YOUR AGE IS WORKING AGAINST YOU

So how'd you get where you're at? Are you like Morris and let your healthy habits slide for a while? Or have you been struggling with your weight for years? If you're honest with yourself, you probably know that you're eating the wrong foods or eating too much overall. And are you really getting after it in the gym...or do you always promise yourself you'll work out and eat right...you know, tomorrow?

While you probably know that your diet and lifestyle aren't as healthy as they could be, there's one more sneaky culprit that may be tipping the scale—your age. If you're over the age of 25, like we are (Morris is 48 and Obi is 41), then your body is working against you. After your mid-20s, your metabolism drops—by 3 to 5 percent each decade.

Slower metabolism = fewer calories burned = more body fat.

If you keep eating the way you did in your 20s, by the time you hit your 40s—or even before—it's easy to pack at least 10 pounds of extra fat on your body. Probably more! That's why most people gain weight as they age. That's what happens when your metabolism slows down, but it can be reversed. In chapter 3, you'll learn about how to jump-start your metabolism and keep it fired up regardless of how old you are. For now, though, let's talk about what makes our program so effective—and unique.

HOW THE CUT IS DIFFERENT

There's no shortage of diet and workout books out there. (If you're like most of the clients that Obi works with, you've probably tried a number of them yourself!) So why create another?

Because The Cut works in the way the others don't. Give us 12 weeks, and you'll shed body fat and increase lean muscle for an overall longer, more toned, healthier look.

Hey, we know you've probably tried to lose weight in the past. But this program isn't like other programs. These factors set The Cut apart from the rest:

■ **It's simple to follow.** Forget diets that insist you consume special shakes or pre-packaged meals, or require you to eat five or six times a day. Some even ask you to follow a liquid diet for a period of time. You'll eat real food—nutritious, filling food—on our program, with most of your calories coming from vegetables, lean protein, fruit, healthy fats, and whole grains.

■ **It's based on the 80/20 rule.** Most strict diets fail because they force you to follow the same rigid rules day after day. If you have one off day or choose to indulge for a special occasion, you've fallen off the program. But The Cut uses the 80/20 diet formula, which means you'll eat healthy and clean 80 percent of the time, indulging in not-so-healthy or cheat meals the other 20 percent of the time. This makes it easier to stick with the diet part of the program—and easier to make a healthy diet like The Cut fit into the real world. After all, what fun is life without the occasional celebration or treat?

■ **It's designed to blast through plateaus.** On most plans you lose weight quickly for a period of time, then—just when you start to feel like the program is really working—bam, you hit a wall. All of a sudden the number on the scale won't budge. The Cut is designed to outsmart your metabolism so that you don't plateau. Yes, you'll lose weight fast during the first three or four weeks on The Cut—but you won't plateau. That's because the Cut program adjusts your daily caloric goal every four weeks to take your new, lower weight into account and to keep the pounds falling off. At the same time, the program is designed to help you build lean muscle from the beginning, which means you burn more calories even as you lose weight (more on how this works in chapter 3). You avoid the dreaded diet plateau where your scale gets stuck for weeks—you'll hit your goal weight more quickly, and you won't get frustrated or lose motivation on the way.

■ **It's balanced.** Ever tried a low-carb or low-fat diet? The rationale behind them is that eliminating a macronutrient like carbs or fat encourages weight loss. (Calories from food come from three macronutrients—carbohydrates, protein, and fat, which we'll explain more on page 23.) Sure, those diets work in the short term, but they're impossible to stick with over time, and even worse, they may be imbalanced so you aren't getting all the nutrients you need. Our program is based on consuming the right balance of carbs, protein, and fat, so you won't have to limit or restrict any of the three macronutrients. That means the program is easier to follow, especially over the long term—and that it's a healthier and more balanced approach to weight loss.

■ **It's customized to you.** This isn't a one-size-fits-all program like many other diets. The number of calories you'll consume depends on your current body weight, and the exercise program is dependent on your current fitness level. Beginners will start doing a more moderate program of strength training and cardio three days a week, while intermediate and advanced exercisers will train more often. Because you can tailor the program to your body and your needs, it will work that much more effectively.

■ **It's designed to build lean muscle.** Many diets focus on food and forget about (or downplay) exercise. That's a huge problem because if you lose weight without exercising, you tend to lose the muscle that keeps your metabolism fired up. That means your metabolism drops, and you need fewer calories than you did before, which often makes for a rebound weight gain. The Cut is based on the latest exercise science and what Obi's learned firsthand training thousands of people. It includes the right amount of exercise in the right order—you'll do weight training first, followed by cardio, which will help you build more lean muscle. Research also shows that this type of exercise helps you maintain your lower, healthier weight after losing extra fat.

■ **It's the right level of intensity.** Our interval-based cardio workouts mean you burn more calories during the workout—and more afterward as well. Unlike some exercise programs that focus on volume or amount of exercise, our program will have you exercising for shorter periods but at higher intensity—for more results in less time!

■ **It's based on your lifestyle.** Do you hate the idea of joining a gym? Or do you travel a lot, so you need flexibility in how to get a workout in? If so, this program is designed with you in mind! You'll find exercise moves you can do at home using your body weight or dumbbells. If you'd rather work out at the gym or health club, you'll find moves that use gym machines and other equipment. Or maybe you want to do both, depending on the day. We've made it easy to fit the plan into your life.

■ **It's not a deprivation diet—you'll get sufficient calories and nutrients.** In order to lose weight, you have to burn more calories than you consume. But too many programs are far too restrictive, which will have you cheating (or quitting) in no time! Our program is different. Because the number of calories you'll consume is determined by your starting body weight, you won't starve. The Cut is based on reasonable caloric restriction, which prevents your metabolism from plummeting. It also means you won't suffer from hunger pangs all day—you'll feel satisfied on the healthy foods The Cut contains.

From Morris:

As an actor, I depend on how I look for part of my livelihood. That doesn't mean it's always easy for me to look the part. One of the challenges of being on set is that there's a constant flow of food. When we get to work, the caterers are there and they'll make anything we want for breakfast—sausages, omelets, French toast, pancakes, whatever we desire. After that, the craft service table will have all the muffins and pastries and doughnuts you can imagine.

A couple of hours after breakfast they'll bring something out like quesadillas for a snack, followed by lunch. Then as soon as lunch is over they put out even more fresh Danishes and other baked goods…and then dinner! We often work 12-, 13-, and 14-hour days, and we're always surrounded by food. In other words, we work long hours and are offered just about every food temptation under the sun.

There's a saying that actors get fat on set. You can see why! Being on set is one of my biggest diet challenges.

Making the Cut: Real People, Real Results

Name: Jeffrey Smith
Age: 36
Location: Fuquay-Varina, North Carolina
Occupation: Plumber
Height: 6'1"
Starting weight: 236 pounds
Ending weight: 196 pounds

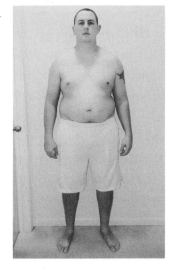

I've wanted to lose weight for the last five or six years. When I joined a gym in 2009, I lost about 20 pounds in a six-month period, then I stopped going—and gained all that weight back plus some more.

I had a long conversation with my wife after I decided to do The Cut—we mutually agreed that I had to give this 110 percent, so I made sure that every day, no matter what, I made the time to go to the gym. She supported me all the way, which made it easier.

The first couple of weeks, the diet was a nightmare for me, though! I couldn't eat fast food or junk food. No cheese, no milk, and no chocolate. But I stayed committed and focused on my goal. I got used to the diet after the first three weeks or so, when I got all that sugar and other bad stuff out of my system and off my mind. Once you get used to your new routine, it comes naturally.

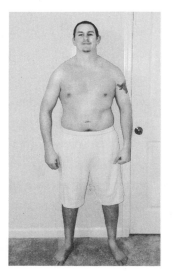

My wife noticed a change in my body about a month into the program—she said I was getting leaner and my arms were toning nicely. I noticed the changes when I first started seeing my two abs about seven weeks in. I haven't seen abs on my body in 20 years! I also *love* to notice my arms filling up my V-neck T-shirts.

I feel like I'm 18 years old again. I feel great. I honestly believe this program helped save my life. I've added 20 years to my life living this new lifestyle—no doubt in my mind!

Now working out is just like the diet—it's just a natural part of my daily lifestyle…and my whole family now goes to the gym each night. My wife has started working out, and my kids enjoy the basketball courts and cardio deck. Exercise is a family activity now and we all love it!

This program is tremendous; if I can do it, anyone can! Take responsibility for your actions and the choices you've made in your life, make a 110 percent commitment to this program, and just do it. I'm the father of six children; work 50 to 60-plus hours per week; and have had double disk back surgery…If I can do this, anyone can. Just commit to it and own it! The Cut gives you

This program is tremendous; if I can do it, anyone can!

every tool you need to be successful. All you have to do is follow the diet, follow the workouts, and give it your best!

From Obi:

Overwhelmed by all the info and claims you see on TV or the Internet? These bogus claims make me nuts. It seems like every day there's some new diet plan or pill or "fat burner" out there claiming to help you shed fat.

The only thing these products will make lighter is your wallet! Trust me, anyone who claims to have found the secret to weight loss is full of it. The only secret is the right diet and the right exercise plan, which you'll find with our program.

GET READY TO GET CUT

You're probably thinking, *Okay, guys, this sounds great, but what exactly does the program look like?* It's simple but phenomenally effective. The diet is a healthy, calorically appropriate plan that is based on your starting body weight and guaranteed to help you smash through weight loss plateaus. We've designed the exercise part of the program to help you burn more calories both during and after your workouts, and build the lean muscle that will rev your metabolism at all times of day.

Curious about how many calories you'll consume? Here's a snapshot:

MEN:	
Starting Weight	*Starting Daily Caloric Intake*
220+ pounds	2,200 to 2,250 calories
180–219 pounds	2,000 to 2,050 calories
160–179 pounds	1,800 to 1,850 calories
Under 160 pounds	1,600 to 1,650 calories

WOMEN:	
Starting Weight	*Starting Daily Caloric Intake*
220+ pounds	1,700 to 1,750 calories
180–219 pounds	1,600 to 1,650 calories
160–179 pounds	1,500 to 1,550 calories
140–159 pounds	1,400 to 1,450 calories
Under 140 pounds	1,300 to 1,350 calories

WHAT ABOUT THE WORKOUT?

Wondering about the workout part of the program? You'll learn more about it in chapters 7 through 14, but here's a sneak peek:

■ **Beginning exercisers.** Don't know your delts from your pecs? You know there's a gym nearby your home or office—but you've never actually set foot in it? Or has it been so long since you worked out that your sneakers have gathered dust? Then you're a beginning exerciser. You will strength-train and do cardio three times a week.

■ **Intermediate exercisers.** If you know you prefer the elliptical to the treadmill, or have a favorite exercise instructor, you're probably already working out several times a week. If that sounds like you, you're an intermediate exerciser on this program. As an intermediate exerciser, you will strength-train and do cardio four times a week.

■ **Advanced exercisers.** Split routines? Tabata training? Power yoga? You've tried it all—or at least you know what those terms mean. If you exercise four times or more a week, you're an advanced exerciser and you will strength-train and do cardio five times a week.

Be honest with yourself about what category you fall into. The goal of The Cut is to get you exercising regularly and following a healthy, clean diet that will help you shed fat. If that means exercising three times a week, as a beginner, that's fine. If it means getting after it five days a week, that's fine, too. In general, the more you exercise, the more quickly you'll lose weight, but we'd rather have you choose a plan that fits your current fitness level and stick to it than try to do more than your body can realistically handle.

For Women Only

When you think of lifting weights, do you picture big sweaty guys grunting and throwing barbells around in the weight room? That's not what this program will have you doing! You can strength-train doing body-weight exercises like modified push-ups, squats, and crunches—or use light dumbbells. You will not be lifting huge, heavy weights and you won't build big, masculine muscles on the Cut program. You will, however, create a lean, toned body that will help you shed fat, speed up your metabolism—and look great naked! Weight training is just as important as cardio and eating clean to lose the fat and maintain those sexy, toned curves, so don't be afraid of the exercise program in this book. It's an essential key to meeting your goals!

Making the Cut: Real People, Real Results

Name: Tiaja Pierre

Age: 45

Location: Denver, Colorado

Occupation: Private investigator

Height: 5'7"

Starting weight: 217 pounds

Ending weight: 187 pounds

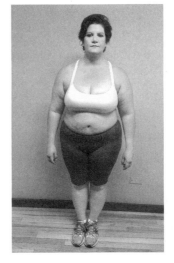

I had always been underweight as a child. However, I gained weight with several pregnancies, and couldn't get it off.

I'd tried other diets and nutritional plans in addition to regularly working out in the past. Initially the plans did work, but life got in the way and other matters took precedence. Plus, some of the plans that I tried when I was younger were fads. I not only gained the weight I lost once I stopped following the plan, but I gained more weight on top of that.

I decided to try The Cut not only because Obi is knowledgeable in his field, but also because I'd seen the kinds of results he gets with this clients. I had high expectations when I started and had confidence that he could help me lose weight. This would be the program that finally worked for me!

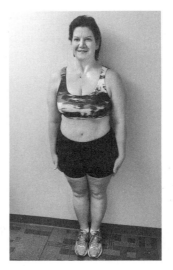

The nutritional part of The Cut was a breeze, but ensuring I had the proper food when traveling or going on business trips required planning in advance. I prepped, cooked, and portioned my food ahead of time and carried it with me on the plane or in the car so I could keep on track nutritionally. I also printed out the meal and workout plans, and put them on index cards. If I was on the road, I looked for grocery stores and asked whether there was a refrigerator and microwave where I'd be staying. And I made sure that they had a health club so I could work out.

The amazing part of the nutrition plan was that I was never hungry and had enough energy to complete each and every workout. I loved that the workouts let me build strength and see my progress, not just in my body and the way it looked, but in the amount of weight I was able to lift. I didn't get

> **I was never hungry and had enough energy to complete each and every workout.**

bulky like some women fear from doing these types of exercises. Though I lost weight, I also lost inches as my body became more compact.

I feel enthusiastic and ecstatic after completing the 12-week Cut. I am starting to see the real me again and welcome the changes that have come from following the plan! It's renewed my faith in myself and my ability to set goals and reach them.

I would strongly encourage anyone who is looking to transform his or her life to try The Cut. This program is for real people who have a life and responsibilities. By putting one foot in front of the other and following the plan properly, results are inevitable, and so is the success you will experience—just as I have!

MENTALLY PREPARE TO CUT

We already said we won't sugarcoat things. The Cut program takes commitment and discipline. Maybe you're worried about whether you can stick with the plan for 12 weeks. Or maybe you wish you could pick up a big bottle of discipline next time you're at the store.

The reality is you can't buy discipline. But you can *build* it just like you build a muscle. In the first few days or weeks, it may be a challenge to make the decisions that will help you shed body fat and keep it off. Keep it up, though, and it will get easier. By the end of the 12 weeks, you'll have transformed not only your body but your mental outlook as well.

Our job is to create an effective plan and help motivate you to follow it. Your job is to work as hard as you can on the Cut program so you can achieve phenomenal results. We believe you can do it. Now it's up to you—to believe in yourself. When you do, you'll not only drop pounds fast, but also develop the skills and embrace the tools you need to get Cut—and to stay Cut—for life.

2 "Eat Carbs, Get Fat"

Debunking Common Fitness Myths

If you see something in print, it must be true? Right? Especially if it's from a well-known fitness celebrity or nutrition expert? Well, you probably know that's not true, but you'd be surprised at how many people fall for common fitness and nutrition myths. In this chapter, we'll set the record straight on what really works and what's just plain fiction.

> **FITNESS MYTH:** Eating small meals throughout the day will speed up your metabolism exponentially and help speed up fat loss.
>
> **FITNESS FACT:** The number of meals you eat doesn't affect your metabolic rate.

Eat more often, jack up your metabolism, right? This fitness "fact" is reported all over the place. Both of us have heard that dozens of times! Well, whoever has ever asserted this should issue a big, fat apology: *I was wrong.*

Your metabolism is much more dependent on your weight, the amount of muscle you have, your gender, your age, and your activity level than how often you eat. Your metabolic rate will not change whether you eat 3 times a day, 6 times a day, or even 10 times a day.

The truth is it's the number of calories you consume, and expend, that determines whether you'll lose weight or gain it. If you consume 2,000 calories, you can spread them among three balanced meals or a bunch of snacks throughout the day and it won't affect your metabolism or whether you lose weight.

However, there is an advantage to eating every four hours or so instead of going longer stretches between meals. Eating more frequently can ease hunger pangs and prevent you from overeating later on. So if you have lunch at noon but won't eat dinner until 7:00 p.m., have a healthy snack at 4:00 or 5:00 p.m. to tide you over until you sit down to eat. This way you'll be able to make healthier choices come dinnertime.

> **FITNESS MYTH:** Eating carbs late at night will make you gain weight.
>
> **FITNESS FACT:** It's the amount of carbs you eat, not the time of day, that matters.

Eat carbs, get fat. That's what many of Obi's clients mistakenly believe, and he has to convince them that their fear of carbs is unfounded. Yet lots of people believe that carbs are more likely to be stored as fat, especially when they're consumed at night.

Want proof? A study published in the *Journal of Obesity* in 2011 divided participants into two groups. Both groups consumed the same calorie-restricted diet that included the same amount of calories, protein, carbs, and fat for six months. One group consumed 80 percent of their carbs late at night while the other consumed them throughout the day.

So the group that ate the carbs at night gained weight, right? Wrong! What may surprise you is that the group that ate their carbs late at night lost significantly more weight and more body fat than the group that consumed their carbs in the daytime! The first group also felt more full and were less hungry during the day than the other group. So eating carbs late at night—as long as you're staying within a healthy number of calories—won't make you fat.

From Morris:

I'm always telling my wife, Pam, she should lift weights, but she's always saying she doesn't want to get big and bulky. She's afraid she'll get huge muscles if she weight-trains and swears she'll "lean out" more if she sticks to the treadmill. What can I say? We've been married for almost 20 years and she still doesn't listen to me!

> **FITNESS MYTH:** Weight training will make women bulk up and look less feminine.
>
> **FITNESS FACT:** Weight training will give women sleek, defined muscles, not bulky ones.

This is a concern that Obi hears all too often from the women he trains. Let us tell you, if you're a woman, lifting weights will not make you bulk up! Even women who weight-train regularly don't produce enough testosterone to develop huge, muscle-bound physiques. The only way a woman can develop that kind of body is to take anabolic steroids, consume lots of extra calories, and train with very heavy weights, like a power lifter. You won't do that on our program.

The bottom line is that lifting weights is integral for body shaping and fat loss. Weight training shapes a woman's body like nothing else. When you lift weights, you add definition to your curves, increase your bone density, improve overall fat loss, increase your energy levels, and even improve the quality of your sleep!

High-intensity strength training—the kind you'll do with our program—will also help you burn more calories after your workout thanks to EPOC, or excess post-exercise oxygen consumption. EPOC is also known as the afterburn effect, and it occurs after high-intensity exercise. On average, EPOC burns an additional 6 to 15 percent of the total calories expended during the workout; the more intense the workout, the higher the EPOC.

Here's more about how EPOC works. Imagine you drive your car for an hour. When you arrive at your destination, you shut off the engine. While the engine is no longer running, it's still warm, and will take some time to cool down. That's what happens after you do an intense workout—your body is still warm afterward. Even after you cool off, your body is still revved for about 24 hours. During that time, it uses extra oxygen

> **FITNESS MYTH:** Eating as little as possible will lead to dramatic weight loss.
>
> **FITNESS FACT:** You have to eat regularly to lose weight; going without food will inhibit weight loss.

to restore itself to homeostasis, a fancy word for its normal resting state. That transition from hot to cold over the next day or so is your body's EPOC response.

This is another big weight loss myth we constantly hear. Eating as little as possible *won't* help you lose weight! When you eat too little, your metabolism drops, which means you burn fewer calories.

You can't outsmart your body. If you're not eating enough, your body knows it's not getting the energy it needs. During times in human history when food was less readily available than it is today, a drastic drop in food intake didn't mean diet, it meant potential starvation. So as a survival mechanism, when you don't eat enough, your metabolism slows down to become more efficient and protect its fat stores—to keep you alive! That means the less you eat, the slower your metabolism becomes—and the more sluggish you feel and the more weight you hold on to.

Research has proven that taking in fewer than 1,200 calories a day produces the largest drop in your RMR, or resting metabolic rate. Besides making you feel exhausted, spacey, and outright crummy, starving yourself is unhealthy. If you try to survive on too few calories for too long, you'll put your body into a catabolic state and lose lean muscle (your body will break it down for energy), which is the biggest driver of your metabolic rate. You'll also be more likely to binge and may set yourself up for more serious health problems like seizures or even a heart attack.

From Morris:

I used to think that the less I ate, the faster I'd lose weight. Before I met Obi, if I had to drop weight for a movie role, I would eat maybe one meal a day and play hours of basketball. I thought the fewer calories I consumed, the better, but my strategy didn't work so well.

I always felt hungry, tired, and off my game. And as I got older, I didn't even lose weight very quickly. I was relieved when Obi explained that eating more, not less, would make me shed weight faster. Now I eat more and I feel better—and look better, too.

FITNESS MYTH: All calories are created equal.

FITNESS FACT: All calories are not created equal.

We all have heard of the old theory "calories in versus calories out" when it comes to weight loss. This can be misleading to the average person who wants to lose weight.

Tracking your calories is important if you want to lose weight because the amount of calories, or energy, you consume will affect whether you gain weight or lose it. You need to eat fewer calories than you burn in order to lose weight. That energy comes from three macronutrients—protein, carbohydrates, and fat—and your body processes these differently. Carbs and fats are used for functional energy, and your body expends less energy to digest and use them. Your body burns off about 5 percent of carb calories during digestion, and about 3 percent of fat calories to digest fat. But your body burns a much higher percentage of calories—20 to 30 percent—to digest protein. This process—expending calories to use them—is called the thermic effect of food.

This doesn't mean you should follow a high-protein diet or any diet that overly emphasizes one type of macronutrient over another. It does mean that you should take in a balance of all three, and make protein a priority with each meal because it's the ultimate MVP, or most valuable player, when it comes to how many calories your body must expend to use it.

> **FITNESS MYTH:** "Fat-burner" supplements can help you lose weight without exercising or changing your diet.
>
> **FITNESS FACT:** There's no magic fat loss or weight loss pill that will, by itself, help you lose weight.

It seems like every day you hear about the latest fat burner or pill that can help you shed body fat. Well, we're sorry to tell you that there's no such thing as a fat-burning pill! The only fat burner—and the most powerful one—is a lifestyle that includes a healthy diet and regular exercise. Because dieting is big business. We have a billion-dollar weight loss industry that pushes miracle pills to people who are desperate to lose weight and want an easy solution. Some supplements, like multivitamins, omega-3 fatty acids, and whey protein, can help you reach your health and fitness goals, but they're no replacement for actual food.

Any supplement company, TV host, or article that claims that its pill or supplement will, on its own, make you lose weight, is lying. Save your money. The only way you can lose body fat for good is by eating healthy and exercising.

The only supplement we recommend is fish oil, because most people don't consume enough healthy fat in the form of omega-3 fatty acids. We also suggest a protein shake post-exercise to help provide your muscles with enough protein to rebuild the damage done during exercise. It's muscle that fuels your metabolism, not a pill.

From Morris:

I confess that I've tried fat burners (supplements that claim to accelerate fat loss) in the past, when I've had to drop weight for a role where I had to take my shirt off. I also tried creatine to try to build muscle. The creatine seemed to help, but I didn't use any supplements when I started working with Obi. I wanted to build as much muscle as I could, so I drank a protein shake before and after my workouts—and got awesome results with no fat burners or any other supplements.

I always drink a chocolate protein shake after my workouts. When I'm really hard-core, I'll even use the shake as a replacement for sweets!

FITNESS MYTH: Doing lots of sit-ups and crunches will eliminate your potbelly and give you washboard, ripped abs.

FITNESS FACT: There's no such thing as spot reduction.

Both men and women crave sculpted, gorgeous abs, so it's understandable to focus on exercises that will target trouble spots. The trouble is, the whole idea of spot reduction is a myth. Exercising your abs won't eliminate the fat on top of them. The only way to remove belly fat is with proper diet and a training regimen that will reduce the fat *all over* your body.

Ab exercises will help build your abdominal muscles, but the only way to make them come out of hibernation is by having a relatively low body fat percentage. Think of the saying, "Abs are made in the kitchen, not the gym." You can do as many crunches as you want, but if you don't eat to reduce body fat then you'll never see them. On average, a woman has to have a body fat percentage of about 15 or lower to have visible abs; a man has to have a body fat percentage of about 12 percent or lower.

FITNESS MYTH: Cardiovascular activity is the best exercise to help you burn calories and shed fat.

FITNESS FACT: A combination of weight training and cardiovascular exercise is the key to burning calories and shedding fat.

Check out any gym and what do you usually see? Far too often, it's women on cardio machines and men in the weight area. Many women avoid lifting weights because they think it will make them bulk up (see page 21) and that all that cardio will burn fat. That's a mistake.

In the meantime, most guys do nothing but lift weights! When a guy asks Obi what he needs to do to get ripped, his response is, "You need to get on that cardio machine and sweat, my friend."

Cardio isn't the answer when it comes to shedding fat—the key is to combine cardio and weight training. Weight training helps you build more lean muscle, which is essential for lasting weight loss. More lean muscle increases your metabolic rate, which means you burn more calories all the time, both in and out of the gym. High-intensity weight training can also produce the EPOC response we talked about earlier in this chapter.

Cardio's advantage is that you typically burn more calories doing cardio than lifting weights. That helps you shed pounds. If you opt for high-intensity cardio (instead of the more moderate intensity most people do), you'll get an EPOC response. It doesn't matter whether you're doing high-intensity weight training or high-intensity cardio—the higher the intensity, the more pronounced the EPOC response.

In short, **weight training + cardio = faster fat loss!** So don't choose cardio or weights—incorporate them both for the results you want.

FITNESS MYTH: It is impossible to cheat on your diet and lose weight at the same time.

FITNESS FACT: You can enjoy a few cheat meals every week—as long as you have a reasonable portion.

You may be surprised that we believe in cheating on an otherwise healthy diet, but we promise you can enjoy a cheat meal several times a week and still lose weight! Eating the same foods day after day can be a drag, and cheat meals are a nice break.

Many nutritionists and fitness experts suggest using the 80/20 or 90/10 rule when it comes to diet. That means eating healthy 80 to 90 percent of the time and indulging 10 to 20 percent of the time. We've found the 80/20 rule more effective than trying to eat clean 90 percent (or even 100 percent!) of the time. Eating healthy and clean five days a week with a cheat meal once or twice a week is a manageable lifestyle. It's also likely to help you meet your weight loss goals—research has proven that too-strict dieting is counterproductive because people are less likely to stick with their plan.

The key to making this work is to watch your portions—the portion size of a cheat meal (or cheat treat) should be about the size of your palm. That's a modest serving (unless you have huge hands like Michael Jordan!).

Making the Cut: Real People, Real Results

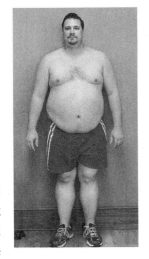

Name: Mike Hopper

Age: 33

Location: Hanover, Indiana

Occupation: Barber

Height: 6'1"

Starting weight: 317.5 pounds

Ending weight: 260 pounds (after the first 12 weeks), 219 pounds after 6 months

Before I started The Cut, I was constantly tired and was in pain every night when I got off work. I was also a ticking time bomb. My blood pressure was 144/88, my cholesterol was 258, and triglycerides were 412. I pretty much only ate junk food and fast food, and very few vegetables. I was constantly in pain; it even hurt to bend over to pick up my shoes in the morning. I was tired all the time and had very bad sleeping habits. I also have suffered from very severe migraines for the past seven years, but I haven't had a migraine since the day I started the program.

After the first 12 weeks on The Cut, my blood pressure was 115/60, my cholesterol was 161, and my triglycerides were 95! My doctor was *very* happy and I feel amazing! My body doesn't hurt like it used to, and I don't have knee or back pain anymore. And it's not a struggle to put my shoes on every morning! I no longer have trouble walking stairs!

It's amazing what a difference 12 weeks of healthy eating and exercise will do. I never ate vegetables before the program and now I eat them every day and actually enjoy them. And I went from being over 100 pounds overweight and doing very little physical activity to having all kinds of energy and feeling great. Sure, I've tried other diet and exercise plans in the past. Everything worked short-term but was almost impossible to follow long-term. This program is different. There is no reason why it won't work for you!

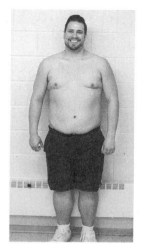

I had more weight to lose, so I decided to follow The Cut for another 12 weeks. From a physical standpoint, it's much easier to work out. When I started, it was hard enough to move on a day-to-day basis, so adding exercise was difficult. Now I can give my workouts 100 percent! Mentally, I'm to the point where there is no question I will reach my goals. I look forward to my workouts now and enjoy eating healthy. It used to be hard eating out with friends when everyone else was eating fried, high-fat foods, and I was eating lean meats, veggies, and plain baked potatoes. Now it doesn't tempt or faze me. I actually want the healthy options now. The lifestyle is ingrained in me.

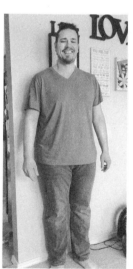

Before I started The Cut, I was constantly tired and was in pain every night when I got off work. After completing the program, I feel amazing. My body doesn't hurt like it used to, and I don't have knee or back pain anymore.

> **FITNESS MYTH:** Drinking coffee is unhealthy because of the caffeine it contains.
>
> **FITNESS FACT:** Drinking coffee is healthy in moderation.

Is coffee bad for you? It depends on which expert you talk to. Too much caffeine (say, more than four or five cups of coffee a day) can cause health issues including insomnia, stomach upset, irritability, nervousness, and muscle tremors.

But caffeine is also a proven performance enhancer athletes have used for years, especially in endurance events. Small amounts of caffeine make you feel more alert and focused, and boost your mood. It may also improve your cardiovascular health—recent research published in the medical journal *Heart* suggests that regular coffee consumption may help reduce your risk of developing heart disease, and other studies suggest that it may reduce your risk of developing type 2 diabetes as well.

Both of us drink coffee with no ill effects on our health or physiques. A cup of coffee can also improve your performance in the gym. Just keep your caffeine intake moderate—about three cups or fewer a day—to avoid stomach issues and trouble sleeping.

From Morris:

Fat makes you fat, right? That's what I always believed, so I was constantly trying to limit my fat intake when I was trying to lose weight. I was surprised Obi suggested I snack on a spoonful of peanut butter or a handful of nuts when I was dieting for *The Best Man Holiday*. I didn't think I could eat fat when I was trying to get Cut. But sometimes that spoonful of peanut butter was the highlight of my day!

Now I make sure to make healthy fat a part of my everyday diet—unsalted almonds are my go-to snack.

> **FITNESS MYTH:** Eating fat will prevent you from losing weight.
>
> **FITNESS FACT:** Fat is good for you, and eating it can help you lose weight.

Let's get this straight, since there's a lot of misinformation out there: Fat is not the demon it's made out to be. As you saw in chapter 1, you get your calories from the three macronutrients—protein, carbohydrates, and fat. Your body needs fat for overall cellular health, for energy, and to absorb vitamins like vitamin A, vitamin D, vitamin E, and vitamin K. Dietary fat also helps you feel full and satisfied longer as it takes longer for the body to digest than carbs. Keeping fat in your diet will help you stick with your diet. Don't be worried about the fact that it contains more calories (9 per gram) than carbs and protein, which both contain 4 per gram. Your body needs some fat for optimal health—and sustainable weight loss!

From a health standpoint, you want to opt for the good fats—monounsaturated and polyunsaturated fats—instead of the bad ones, saturated fats and trans-fatty acids. Good sources of monounsaturated fats include olive oil, avocados, peanut butter, and canola oil.

The polyunsaturated fats are omega-3 fatty acids and omega-6 fatty acids. Good sources of omega-3 fatty acids include fatty fish (including salmon, herring, and trout), walnuts, flaxseeds, sunflower seeds, and corn oil. Corn oil, soybean oil, and other plant-based vegetable oils are all good sources of omega-6 fatty acids.

Eating moderate amounts of monounsaturated and polyunsaturated fats helps you lower your bad cholesterol, raise your good cholesterol, reduce blood pressure, and lower your triglycerides, or the amount of sugar you have circulating in your blood. (High triglycerides are linked to a higher risk of heart disease.) Both omega-3 and omega-6 fats also help reduce your risk of heart disease and stroke.

Limit saturated fat, which is found in red and fattier meat, eggs, poultry, and dairy products; excessive saturated fat has been linked with health conditions like high blood pressure, high cholesterol, heart disease, stroke, and type 2 diabetes. (You can still eat meat—just choose lean cuts, which contain a lower percentage of fat.) You should avoid trans-fatty acids, or partially hydrogenated oils, which are found in fried foods and baked goods like cookies and cakes. Research suggests that trans-fatty acids appear to be even worse for your health than saturated fats, so we suggest you eliminate them from your diet, except perhaps for the occasional cheat meal or treat.

So now that you know the truth—and science—behind common fitness and nutrition myths, let's get into the science of your metabolism. In the next chapter, you'll learn all about what your metabolism is, what it does, why it slows down, and the different ways you can speed it up.

3 Accelerate Your Metabolism

Why Yours Is Slow—and How to Speed It Up

Ever envied people you know who seem to be able to eat whatever they want without ever putting on a pound? Hey, we do, too! Those effortlessly lean people often have high metabolisms that keep them trim—without spending a lot of time in the gym.

But what exactly is metabolism, anyway? What determines whether it's fast or slow? If yours is slow, are you cursed forever? (Don't worry—you're not!) Understanding how your metabolism functions, and how to change it, is *the* key to shedding body fat. You'll discover why in this chapter.

From Morris:

Before I started working with Obi, I didn't really understand how my metabolism worked. I knew I couldn't eat like I did in my 20s without gaining weight, but I didn't realize that my metabolism—not just what I was eating—was the culprit.

I didn't just lose weight during the 12 weeks I worked with Obi—I added lean muscle. My chest, back, and arms all got bigger, and that extra muscle fired up my metabolism and keeps it running hot. That means I'm burning more calories all the time, even if I have a 14-hour day on set and can't work out.

UNDERSTANDING YOUR METABOLISM

It's natural to assume that someone who's ripped or never seems to have weight issues has a fast metabolism. But we both know people who look fantastic because they maintain super-strict diets and work out hard nearly every day of the week. So don't assume that a speedy metabolism is the only reason the person looks so great.

That said, people love to blame their metabolisms for being overweight. "It's not my fault," they say. "I have a slow metabolism." Or, "Even when I diet, I can't lose weight. My metabolism is sluggish."

Even if that's the case, that slow or sluggish metabolism is a result not of their genetics but rather of their lifestyle choices, which we'll talk more about in a bit.

Fast metabolism. Slow metabolism. So what exactly does *metabolism* mean? We don't have to get all scientific here. The simplest way to explain is that **metabolism is the process of converting what you eat and drink into energy to fuel your body.** This process takes a certain amount of energy, or calories. The amount of calories that your body uses for its most basic functions (like breathing) is called your basal, or resting, metabolic rate, or BMR.

Well, obviously you do a lot more in a typical day than breathe! In addition to the calories you burn through your BMR, you expend calories during the day whether you're working, walking, exercising, or simply sitting on the couch watching *Rosewood*. You also burn some calories when you digest food, which is called the thermic effect of food.

So your metabolism in total—the amount of calories you'll burn in a typical day—is dependent on three things: your basal metabolic rate; the amount of activity you do during the day; and the food you eat (but not how often you eat, as you saw in the last chapter). The biggest factor is your BMR, which makes up about 70 percent of your total metabolism.

Your BMR depends on the following:

- Your size. Simply put, if you're 6'2", you're going to burn more calories, on average, than someone who's 5'6". The heavier you are, the more calories you burn all the time.

- Your gender. In general, men tend to have more lean muscle mass and less body fat than women. That means their metabolic rates tend to be higher than women's.

- Your muscle mass. The more muscle you have, the higher your metabolic rate will be.

- Your age. As you get older, you tend to lose muscle, which slows your metabolic rate.

Take a look at these factors, and what becomes obvious? The only factor within your control is the amount of muscle you have. You can't grow another 6 inches and you definitely can't turn back the clock. But you can keep your BMR elevated by building and retaining muscle.

Most people fail to do the kind of exercise that lets them retain muscle, however. Remember that after you reach the age of 30, you start to lose lean muscle mass at a rate of between 3 and 8 percent per decade, which causes a 3 to 5 percent drop in metabolic rate each decade. You lose muscle, your metabolic rate drops, and you begin to gain body fat, and gain weight as well. (The amount of fat you have is your body fat percentage; your weight is the number you see on the scale.)

People often assume that a slowing metabolism is a normal part of getting older, but we're here to tell you that's not the case! The good news is that lifestyle factors play a bigger role. In other words, you're in charge. Now, if you live a sedentary lifestyle, your metabolism will drop. The more time you spend on your butt sitting on the couch, the slower your metabolism will be.

From Morris:

If you want to change your body, the question is: How badly do you want it? It's like being in the acting business. Everyone wants to be a star—but no one wants to do the work! It's the same with changing your body—you have to be willing to do the work.

EXERCISE IS THE METABOLIC ANSWER

So what's the answer? Exercise—specifically, the right kind of exercise. That's the only way to preserve your lean muscle mass, which is the driver of your metabolism.

People have different roadblocks when it comes to exercise. Some people simply aren't working out at all, and they need to be encouraged to develop a regular routine. But what if you do exercise, yet don't see many results? We bet you're exercising wrong.

You already know that in general women prefer cardio and men prefer lifting weights, but that's not the only issue with exercise. You need a workout plan that includes two vital elements—strength training, or weight lifting, and cardiovascular exercise. That's the type of training you'll do with our program. The Cut is designed to put more lean muscle on your body, which will increase your metabolic rate and turn your body into a blazing-hot furnace that burns more calories all the time. That's a beautiful thing.

You already know that strength training helps build and maintain lean muscle. That's only half of the exercise equation, though. The other is cardio—but not just any cardio. Low- or moderate-intensity cardio exercise is better than no exercise at all, but neither does a lot to maintain lean muscle or impact your metabolism. High-intensity cardio like sprinting, boxing, soccer, and plyometrics also helps maintain lean muscle and prevent age-related metabolic decline.

From Obi:

Don't blame your genetics for your body. You can overcome bad genetics with the right diet and exercise program.

From Morris:

Mainly I work out in the morning. Sometimes if I have a long shooting day, I'll go to the gym at three thirty or four in the morning. Some days are too intense for me to get it in and I'll miss a day, but I try to work out at least two days a week during the week and then I get it in on the weekends, too. The closer it gets to a scene or show where I have to take my shirt off, the more cardio I do!

We realize that not everyone can do high-intensity workouts like running or playing basketball all the time. They can be hard on your body and joints, especially high-impact activities like sprinting and plyometrics. But you don't have to do long sessions of high-intensity cardio to reap its benefits. Even short bursts of high-intensity effort, called interval training, will help you preserve lean muscle mass, increase fat loss, and speed up your metabolism. Another huge benefit of high-intensity exercise is that it cuts your workout time—you can burn as many calories in half the time as you would if you did lower-intensity activities.

The following activities can all be high-intensity:

- Basketball (Morris's favorite workout!)
- Boxing/kickboxing
- Circuit training (weight lifting done with no rests during sets)
- Cycling (indoor or outdoor)
- Plyometrics (jumping or explosive power moves, including jumping rope)
- Rowing
- Running
- Soccer
- Swimming
- Tennis

All of these activities continuously use many muscle groups, which elevates your heart rate and burns a lot of calories. When you perform high-intensity exercise, you use more muscle fibers overall, which helps produce an EPOC response that will burn additional calories post-workout. Your effort matters; if you want to build and maintain lean muscle, you need to challenge yourself beyond what feels comfortable. But don't worry—you'll choose a program that fits your fitness level and individual needs.

That high-intensity exercise means that you burn more calories than you normally would while you're doing it, and afterward. Plus, it's helping you keep that lean muscle. So from a metabolic and calorie-burning standpoint, it's win/win/win. The more calories you burn through the kind of high-intensity exercise you'll do with our program, the higher you'll ratchet up your BMR.

From Morris:

When I first saw how ripped Obi was, I was impressed. I know how hard it is to look like that as you get older. I figured he must be taking supplements or fat burners to look the way he does, and that he'd want me on some of that stuff, too.

Well, as soon as I started talking with Obi I realized he didn't use fat burners or supplements other than protein powder and fish oil. He was legit—a top-notch, highly conditioned athlete who broke many track sprinting school records when at Cal State Fullerton University.

Obi is 100 percent natural, as they say in the bodybuilding business. That means he doesn't use steroids or other drugs to put on muscle. I've never used steroids, either, and I wanted to work with someone who's legit. Obi built his body and helps others build theirs the healthy, drug-free way, and that's a big reason I chose to work with him.

From Obi:

Morris is right—I believe you should, and can, build your best body the natural way through proper diet and the right kind of exercise. I've been a fitness professional for more than 13 years now. I've appeared on magazine covers and been featured as a fitness expert for more than seven years, and I have *never* taken an illegal drug or used steroids. I strongly recommend against using unproven supplements to change your body. The best supplement to take? Healthy, clean, whole food.

Making the Cut: Real People, Real Results

Name: Rome Douglas
Age: 39
Location: Upland, California
Occupation: Retired professional football player; currently sales manager for industrial packaging supplies company
Height: 6'7"
Starting weight: 385 pounds
Ending weight: 353.6 pounds

I recognized that I needed help with my weight as I was approaching 400 pounds. I decided to follow The Cut because I've known Obi for years and trusted him to create a program that would work—and be good for my body.

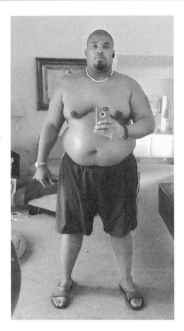 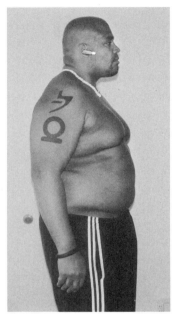

Initially it was hard to stick with the diet part of the program—I felt jittery and slightly irritable because my body and mind were conditioned to fill up my plate every time I ate. But I realized I was eating out of habit and stuck with the diet. I've not only lost a ton of weight in a short amount of time—I also have a ton of energy. I feel like I did when I was playing sports!

I like The Cut because it's also helped me develop healthy habits that I can keep for life.

I like The Cut because it's also helped me develop healthy habits that I can keep for life.

BETTER METABOLISM IN A BOTTLE? NOT SO FAST

You know now that the way to a faster metabolism is one word—*muscle*. But that's not what many supplement companies would have you believe. Even though you learned last chapter that there's no such thing as a fat-burner pill, the weight loss supplement industry would have you believe otherwise. You're constantly bombarded with claims and advertisements about the latest breakthrough pill or supplement that claims to help you lose weight, get ripped, or increase your metabolism.

So why do people fall for these products? First, it's normal to want to find the easy way out. There's also probably no fitness subject that is as confusing to the average person as metabolism. Remember that lots of people believe, wrongly, that eating six or seven small meals a day will speed up your metabolism. Well, another common myth is that there are foods or supplements that will boost your metabolism.

Don't feel bad if you've spent money on "proven" supplements that did a whole lot of nothing when it came to losing weight. After all, it seems like every month or so you hear about a new supplement, plant, or herb that's supposed to help you lose weight. So let's take a closer look at the evidence—the published research and the opinion of the National Institutes of Health (NIH), an objective government agency that has no financial interest in any of these products—regarding these products:

- **Bitter orange.** *The Claim:* This stimulant is found in some weight loss supplements and is supposed to suppress appetite, burn more calories, and increase the breakdown of fat. *The Verdict:* According to the NIH, it may have an effect on resting metabolic rate, but it's not clear whether taking bitter orange affects weight loss. *The Bad News:* It can cause side effects like an increase in heart rate and blood pressure, chest pain, and anxiety.
- **Caffeine.** *The Claim:* Caffeine is found in many weight loss supplements, presumably because research shows that it does help to break down fat. *The Verdict:* The NIH states that caffeine has a *possible* modest effect on weight loss. *The Bad News:* Taking too much of it (more than 400 milligrams/day—about the amount in four regular cups of coffee) can cause anxiety, jitters, upset stomach, nausea, and other side effects, and we don't recommend taking it in a supplement form.
- **Calcium.** *The Claim:* There is research to suggest that consuming calcium may help you lose weight, especially if you don't consume enough of it. *The Verdict:* The National Institutes of Health states, "Most studies have found that calcium—from foods or dietary supplements—has little if any effect on body weight and amount of body fat."
- **Chromium.** *The Claim:* Chromium is a mineral that is claimed to help build muscle and create fat loss. *The Verdict:* Research is mixed; the NIH concludes that some

studies suggest chromium may produce a small weight loss. However, most of those studies were conducted with a small number of people over a brief period of time. In other words, the jury's still out.

- **Chili peppers.** *The Claim:* Some studies have found that eating chili peppers can briefly boost metabolism and may also help produce fat loss due to their capsaicinoids, the substances that make the peppers taste spicy. *The Verdict:* It's way too early for researchers to recommend that you eat a certain amount of chili peppers each day for lasting weight loss!

- **Conjugated linoleic acid, or CLA.** *The Claim:* Supposedly, this supplement can reduce body fat. *The Verdict:* According to the NIH, CLA has minimal effect on body fat and body weight. *The Bad News:* CLA can cause abdominal pain and discomfort, constipation, diarrhea, and upset stomach.

- **Garcinia cambogia.** *The Claim:* There are claims that this supplement helps suppress your appetite, decrease the number of fat cells your body makes, and produce weight loss. *The Verdict:* Research on this supplement is inconclusive, and the NIH states that garcinia cambogia has little to no effect on weight loss. *The Bad News:* This supplement may cause side effects like headaches and nausea.

- **Green tea/green tea extract.** *The Claim:* Some studies have found that green tea and green tea extract can temporarily boost your metabolic rate. *The Verdict:* Review studies that look at most of the published research have found this increase is short-lived, and not enough to create any significant weight loss. *The Bad News:* While green tea is generally healthy, green tea extract can cause side effects including nausea, constipation, and high blood pressure; it may also cause liver damage in some people.

- **Guar gum.** *The Claim:* This is soluble dietary fiber that is supposed to make you feel fuller and prevent weight gain. *The Verdict:* Published research has found no proven effect on body weight. *The Bad News:* Guar gum may cause abdominal pain, nausea, diarrhea, cramps, and flatulence.

- **Pyruvate.** *The Claim:* Often found in weight loss supplements, pyruvate is claimed to reduce body fat. *The Verdict:* The NIH's position is that it has a *possible* minimal effect on weight loss.

- **Raspberry ketone.** *The Claim:* This is a relatively new supplement that claims to be a powerful fat burner. *The Verdict:* According to the NIH, raspberry ketone has not been studied enough to determine whether it has any effect on body fat or weight loss. *The Bad News:* The NIH has yet to determine whether it's even safe to take.

■ **Yohimbe.** *The Claim:* Found in many weight loss supplements, this herb is supposed to increase weight loss. *The Verdict:* After reviewing the published research, the NIH has stated that yohimbe has no effect on weight loss. *The Bad News:* It's also considered unsafe and can cause high blood pressure, anxiety, headaches, heart attack, heart failure, or even death.

From Obi:

Educating you about supplements is a topic of personal importance to me as I've had at least a dozen supplement companies ask me to serve as their spokesperson. I've turned down every one. I will never sacrifice my credibility to make an extra dollar and I will never say a product does something that it doesn't! That's a big reason I wanted to write this book with Morris—I want to help prevent you from spending boatloads of money on weight loss products that don't work and to help you get in the best shape possible the healthy way.

If these supplements actually did what they claim, two-thirds of Americans wouldn't be overweight or obese! Weight loss supplements always seem to claim the same thing—they'll help you break down fat! They'll speed up your metabolism! They'll suppress your appetite! They'll expedite fat loss! The claims may be impressive, but the reality is that most supplements have little impact on fat loss, metabolism, or anything else. By themselves, they don't help you accelerate your metabolism or lose weight any faster or magically break down your fat stores or eliminate belly fat. There are a few supplements that can be beneficial (like omega-3 fatty acid supplements), provided you're exercising and eating right. Supplements are meant to assist your diet and exercise program, not replace it.

Whenever a doctor, fitness expert, nutritionist, researcher, or anyone else makes a blanket or controversial statement about losing weight, you should be on your guard. Don't accept that information as gospel. Do your own research, and then form your opinion about it. Even the most credible experts are human and make mistakes. In short, if something sounds too good to be true when it comes to helping you boost your metabolism, lose weight, or shed body fat, it probably is.

Hopefully you've learned from this chapter that the only proven way to increase your metabolism is with the proper type and amount of exercise—specifically strength training and high-intensity cardio, which will help you build and retain the lean muscle that will boost your metabolism. Now that you know the *why*, let's move on to the *how*: the diet that will help you lose body weight and fat, and the exercises and workouts that will enable you to keep your metabolism firing on high.

Part Two

Eat to Get Cut

In the following three chapters, you'll learn how to eat while on The Cut. Chapter 4 gives you the blueprint for the basic meal plan and explains why it's so effective. You'll find the actual Cut meal plans in chapter 5. Chapter 6 includes delicious, simple Cut recipes.

4 The Basics of the Cut Meal Plans

Eating to Shed Fat and Boost Energy

Your diet—what you eat, and how much—is critical to your success on The Cut. In this chapter, you'll learn about the basics of the Cut meal plans. In chapter 5, you'll find the specific meal plans, which will depend on your current body weight:

MEN:	
Starting Weight	*Starting Daily Caloric Intake*
220+ pounds	2,200 to 2,250 calories
180–219 pounds	2,000 to 2,050 calories
160–179 pounds	1,800 to 1,850 calories
Under 160 pounds	1,600 to 1,650 calories

WOMEN:	
Starting Weight	*Starting Daily Caloric Intake*
220+ pounds	1,700 to 1,750 calories
180–219 pounds	1,600 to 1,650 calories
160–179 pounds	1,500 to 1,550 calories
140–159 pounds	1,400 to 1,450 calories
Under 140 pounds	1,300 to 1,350 calories

The meal plans are designed to provide you enough calories from healthy, clean foods so you'll feel satisfied during the day, while allowing you to lose a minimum of 1 or 2 pounds per week. The balance of proteins, carbs (both starchy carbs and fibrous carbs, which we'll talk about in a bit), and healthy fat should prevent you from feeling hungry between meals—that's what the people who participated in our focus group told us! If you do get hungry between meals, drink more water, or snack on a handful of raw broccoli, peppers, or carrots. They'll fill you up without a lot of extra calories.

On each plan, you'll consume the same average number of calories a day for the first four weeks. During the next four weeks (week 5 to week 8), your daily calorie intake will drop slightly; during the last four weeks (week 9 to week 12), your calorie intake will drop again. This caloric reduction takes into account the weight you've already lost on the program, and will keep you from hitting a plateau where you stop losing weight.

THE CUT DIET

The Cut is based on natural, whole foods that are loaded with nutrients and fiber that will help stave off hunger while giving you steady energy all day. While the calorie totals of the plans vary, each plan is based on the four following components:

- **Lean protein:** Lean protein at every meal, to help create and maintain lean muscle.
- **Starchy carbs:** Healthy complex carbs (what we'll call starchy carbs) for energy and satisfaction.
- **Fibrous carbs:** A variety of vegetables and fruits (what we'll refer to as fibrous carbs) for energy, vitamins, and fiber.
- **Healthy fats:** Healthy fats to help your body absorb certain nutrients and feel satisfied.

To make things simple to follow, we've calculated the number of servings of each of these four components that you'll eat each day, based on your gender and starting body weight.

For example, if you're a 5'2" woman whose starting weight is 138 pounds, during the first four weeks on the plan, each day you'll consume:

- 4 servings of lean protein;
- 2 servings of starchy carbs;
- 4 servings of fibrous carbs; and
- 3 servings of healthy fats.

And if you're a 5'8" man whose starting weight is 228 pounds, during the first four weeks on the plan, each day you'll consume:

- 7 servings of lean protein;
- 6 servings of starchy carbs;
- 5 servings of fibrous carbs; and
- 6 servings of healthy fats.

The Cut diet plans emphasize eating lean protein and vegetables. While these plans are based on consuming a certain number of calories, you needn't count calories to succeed. You just follow the number of portions, swapping in different foods as you'd like. We've provided you with some sample daily plans to give you some ideas, but they're only a guideline. The "Cut Food Lists" below let you swap different foods, depending on what you feel like eating. You'll also find recipes that meet the Cut program guidelines in chapter 6.

Portion sizes are really important. Not only do most people choose the wrong kinds of foods—they also eat far too much of them! We've made it easy for you by giving suggested portions for each food you'll eat. Not only will this keep your calories in the suggested range, you'll also relearn the appropriate portion sizes. As you start to eat healthy foods that nourish your body, provide energy, and support weight loss, you won't have to battle the same kinds of cravings that can sabotage so many typical diets. And as your stomach becomes used to consuming smaller amounts of food, you'll find that you're satisfied with smaller portions. Many of our focus group participants told us they couldn't believe how much smaller their meals became—yet they still felt full! Why? First, protein takes longer to digest; second, the healthy carbs you eat help fill you up and keep you feeling full for hours. This will help you maintain your weight long after you've completed The Cut!

Finally, you'll also consume a whey protein shake five days a week on the Cut program (see recipe, page 60). Drink it an hour before you work out, and whenever you prefer on days you don't exercise. The shake will give you extra energy and protein to help build and retain the lean muscle that drives your metabolism. We also suggest you take fish oil supplements to increase your intake of healthy omega-3 fats while on The Cut. The fish oil counts as a healthy fat on the program. (If you don't want to take fish oil, that's fine—swap in one serving of healthy fat instead.) Finally, we recommend a multivitamin to make sure that you're getting essential vitamins and minerals.

Making the Cut: Real People, Real Results

Name: Olivia Rose Bolton
Age: 24
Location: San Antonio, Texas
Occupation: Full-time student and mother
Height: 5'2"
Starting weight: 172.4 pounds
Ending weight: 144 pounds

Ever since giving birth to my daughter, who's now a toddler, I've struggled with my weight. I had success with one diet, but I had to make special meals that were different from what I made for my family. That was unrealistic for me. I like that on The Cut, the meals are something my whole family can enjoy.

> I had success with one diet, but I had to make special meals that were different from what I made for my family. That was unrealistic for me. On The Cut, the meals are something my whole family can enjoy.

I wasn't sure what my husband would think of the meals because of how we normally ate before I did the program—I made a lot of pasta, casseroles, and other heavy dishes—but he loved how simple yet flavorful the meals were. He was happy we could still have pasta, sweet potatoes, and brown rice; just the portions, sauces, and dressings changed. I was able to find a healthier way to cook without adding sauces, salt, and calories to everything.

I felt a difference in my body during the first week of The Cut. Not only did I lose 5 pounds in five days, but I was starting to feel more energetic and not so sluggish. I was definitely sore but it was a good feeling! The strength training was my favorite part of the program.

I had the misconception that women who lifted weights would start to look masculine. Boy, was I wrong! Strength training is what made me more defined and got me pumped to tackle the cardio. I noticed a huge difference in my arms specifically using the strength training, and compliments have been pouring in.

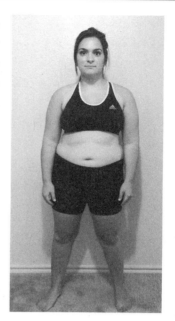

The interval training, or sprinting at 6 mph then walking at 3 mph at 30-second intervals, got my heart rate up, but I didn't feel like I was killing myself on the treadmill. I noticed after a while that I wasn't getting as winded as I did before, and I could increase my sprints to 7 mph. After 12 weeks, I feel more confident, energetic, and like I have my old spark back. I can finally run without feeling like I'm going to pass out, and I feel stronger than ever.

My toddler picks up on everything I do, and I hated that she saw that Mommy ate so unhealthy and couldn't keep up with her without getting winded. Now my daughter will randomly try to do squats and

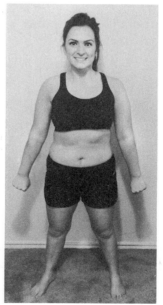

push-ups when she sees Mommy doing them at the park. She has gotten so used to me going to the gym every night that like clockwork, she brings me my tennis shoes and shaker cup, saying "Mommy go gym?" That feels fantastic—knowing your child sees you working hard and that you're setting the example of a healthy lifestyle.

The Cut has completely changed how I think about nutrition and exercise. It's also helped my personal life because I now have the confidence and energy to be a better wife and mother. I'm grateful for this experience and my newfound passion for living a healthy lifestyle!

THE CUT SERVINGS CHART

As we explained, the number of servings of the four food groups you'll consume depends on your target number of calories. In most cases, that caloric target will drop every four weeks to help avoid weight loss plateaus. Here are the number of servings you'll have depending on your target calorie intake:

	Number of Servings/Day								
Daily Caloric Target	*1,200*	*1,300*	*1,400*	*1,500*	*1,600*	*1,700*	*1,800*	*2,000*	*2,220*
Lean protein (P)	4	4	4	4	5	5	5	6	7
Starchy carbs (SC)	2	3	3	3	3	4	5	5	6
Fibrous carbs (C)	4	4	5	5	5	5	5	5	5
Healthy fats (F)	3	3	3	4	4	4	5	6	6

Portion Sizes: How Big Should They Be?

We've listed the amount of food you should eat in the diet plan, but you may not always have access to a food scale and/or measuring cups—and you really don't need them if you learn a few simple tricks. Here is a simple guide for what portion sizes look like for each of the types of food you'll eat on the Cut diet plan:

Food	Serving Size	Estimate
Proteins	3 ounces	Palm of your hand
Starchy carbs (not fruits/vegetables)	4 ounces/½ cup	Handful
Vegetables (except for leafy greens)	8 ounces/1 cup	One fist
Leafy vegetables	16 ounces/2 cups	Two fists
Fruits	8 ounces/1 cup	One fist
Healthy fats (butters and oils)	2 teaspoons	Half your thumb
Healthy fats (nuts and seeds)	1 ounce/⅛ cup	Your thumb

Note: A typical serving of protein is 3 ounces, but for lunches and dinners Monday through Friday of all 12 weeks on the plan, you'll consume 2 servings, or 6 ounces, of a lean protein.

A Sample Cut Meal Plan

In the next chapter, you'll find the Cut meal plans for men and women of different body weights. Each plan is divided into three sections of four weeks each: week 1 through week 4; week 5 through week 8; and week 9 through week 12. During each four-week section, you'll consume the same basic diet Monday through Friday, with cheat meals on Saturday and Sunday. Here's the week 1 through week 4 Cut diet plan for a man who weighs more than 220 pounds (with a daily goal of 2,200 calories). He'll consume 7 servings of lean protein; 6 servings of starchy carbs; 5 servings of fibrous carbs; and 6 servings of healthy fats.

Here's what a typical day on the plan might look like:

Morning (or before working out)
  Protein shake (P)

Breakfast
  2 eggs, cooked any way (2 P)
  1 cup cooked oatmeal, plain (2 SC)
  1 banana (C)
  2 fish oil capsules (F)

Lunch
  6 ounces chicken breast, chopped (2 P)
  1 cup black beans (2 SC)
  4 cups spinach-and-kale mix (2 C)
  2 teaspoons olive oil (F)

Snack
  ¼ cup unsalted almonds (about 24 almonds) (2 F)

Dinner
  Carne Asada Tacos (2 servings) (see recipe, page 102) (2 P 2 SC 2 F)
  2 cups steamed broccoli or mixed vegetables (2 C)

THE CUT FOODS

The Cut meal plan is designed to keep your metabolism revved with plenty of protein and nutrients from complex carbohydrates, vegetables and fruits, and a little bit of healthy fat. Each day's plan is a blueprint—you can follow it as is, or swap in other allowed foods from the same category, as long as you keep the portions the same.

The way you prepare your food is also important. Use cooking methods like grilling, braising, baking, or roasting that add a minimal amount of fat to your food. Fat—even healthy fat—contains a lot of calories (9 calories per gram) compared with protein and carbs (which each contain 4 calories per gram), so you want to be mindful of your portions when eating foods like nuts and olive oil. Use a measuring spoon until you're sure you can serve yourself the correct amount.

The Cut Food Lists

Proteins (P)

A serving is 3 ounces of the following:

Beef (any lean cut)

Chicken

Eggs and/or egg whites (1 egg = 1 serving; 5 egg whites = 1 serving)

Fish (including haddock, salmon, swordfish, tilapia, whitefish)

Lobster

Low-fat or no-fat cottage cheese (½ cup = 1 serving)

Low-fat or nonfat Greek yogurt (Greek yogurt contains more protein than regular yogurt; ½ cup = 1 serving)

Pork (lean cuts)

Shrimp

Tempeh

Tofu (firm or soft)

Tuna (canned, packaged, or fresh)

Turkey

Starchy Carbs (SC)

A serving is ½ cup of the following:

Beans/legumes (for example, black beans, kidney beans, garbanzo beans, white beans)
Bread (whole-grain or multigrain preferred; 1 slice is a serving)
Farro
Millet
Oatmeal (plain)

Oats, rolled
Pasta (whole-grain preferred)
Potatoes (any type)
Quinoa
Rice (brown preferred)
Sweet potatoes
Tortillas (whole-grain or corn)

Fibrous Carbs (C)

Vegetables

A serving of non-leafy vegetables is 1 cup; a serving of leafy vegetables is 2 cups.

Alfalfa sprouts
Artichokes
Asparagus
Bean sprouts
Broccoli
Brussels sprouts
Cabbage
Carrots
Cauliflower

Celery
Corn
Cucumbers
Garlic
Green beans
Kale
Mushrooms
Onions
Peas (any kind)

Peppers (all types, including hot)
Radishes
Scallions
Spinach
Squash (all types)
Swiss chard
Tomatoes
Water chestnuts

Fruits

A serving is 1 cup or 1 medium whole fruit.

Apples
Apricots

Avocados
Bananas

Cantaloupe
Cranberries

Grapefruit	Peaches	Raisins
Grapes	Pears	Strawberries
Honeydew melon	Pineapple	Watermelon
Oranges	Plums	

Healthy Fats (F)

A serving is 2 teaspoons of the nut butters and oils; a serving is also ⅛ cup (2 tablespoons) of nuts or seeds.

Almond butter	Olive oil	Pistachios (unsalted)
Almonds (unsalted)	Olives (all types)	Sesame seeds
Canola oil	Peanut butter	Sunflower oil
Coconut oil	Peanuts (unsalted)	Sunflower seeds
Flaxseeds/flaxseed oil	Pecans (unsalted)	Walnuts (unsalted)

Fruits Versus Vegetables: Does It Matter?

On The Cut, fruits and vegetables fall into the same group—fibrous carbs. While fruits usually contain more calories per serving than vegetables, both contain essential vitamins, and you should eat both on the plan. Vegetables provide more bulk and fiber calorie for calorie, and will help you feel full and satisfied. But fruit can help satisfy your sweet tooth. You'll have at least one serving of fibrous carbs at each meal, which will also get you in the habit of including them in your diet even after you complete The Cut.

Making the Cut: Real People, Real Results

Name: Will Capello
Age: 32
Location: Gonzales, Louisiana
Occupation: Process operator
Height: 5'11"
Starting weight: 230 pounds
Ending weight: 197 pounds

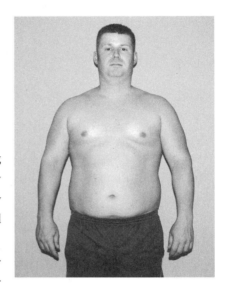

I have struggled with my weight for as long as I can remember, and this time I was at my all-time heaviest. When I had to order new work pants in a bigger size, I drew the line and decided to do something.

I've always ridden that infamous metabolic yo-yo. I'd lose 30 pounds, get to looking and feeling good, and then totally lose momentum. Then I'd be back to square one. That was very stressful mentally.

I've tried all kinds of diets and eating tricks. Low-carb was the one I typically used the most. The diets worked for short periods of time but I would get so burned out eating the same stuff. I just had no variety and felt like I was depriving myself. Then, when I came off the diet, all that hard work would go down the drain, and I was back trying to get the weight back down. I just hadn't been able to figure out a diet and exercise plan that worked well with my lifestyle.

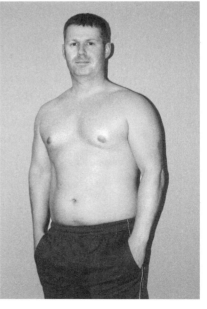

The main issue I dealt with on The Cut was that urge to eat other foods that weren't on the diet—you know, like that big plate of spaghetti and meatballs, pizza, beans and rice with sausage and gumbo. For me it was a matter of telling myself no.

I drank plenty of water to try to stay full so I wouldn't crave anything and tried to avoid situations where I would be tempted to eat off the program. Even though it took discipline, I enjoyed the diet more than other diets. I loved this diet because you can eat a variety of good foods and not feel so deprived. Plus, I always had energy.

> I loved this diet because you can eat a variety of good foods and not feel so deprived. Plus, I always had energy.

At first on The Cut, it was just mentally taxing knowing I had a long way to go to get in great shape. But after a few weeks, I felt excellent. I had more energy and was seeing progress. The foods are clean but tasty, and are something I can eat every day. The workouts are intense, but I really feel good after a gym session.

The most challenging part was staying consistent with the cardio. I've done lots in the past but never this consistently. It was just mind over matter for me. I just kept my rock music blaring on my iPhone and kept pushing through.

By about the end of the first month, my pants were feeling looser and I had more energy. I was getting stronger in the gym and had more stamina. After 12 weeks, I feel great. I'm going to continue working out to get beach-ready for next summer!

From Obi:

You will eat carbs on this program. Carbs are not evil! They're energy your body needs—just like gas to a car. Without gas, your car won't run. Without carbs, your brain and body won't have the energy you need to get through the day. The American Dietetic Association recommends at least 130 grams of carbs per day to meet basic energy needs and to supply enough glucose for your brain to function optimally.

THE IMPORTANCE OF CHEAT MEALS

During every week of The Cut, you'll follow the same basic diet Monday through Friday. On Saturday and Sunday, however, you'll eat two cheat meals each, for a total of four cheat meals each weekend. You can "cheat" with whatever foods you love, including the following:

- Bacon/sausage (or other fatty meats)
- Doughnuts
- Enchiladas
- French fries
- Fried chicken
- Hamburger
- Ice cream
- Pancakes/waffles
- Pastrami sandwich
- Pizza
- Subway sandwich

Cheat meals play an important role in the Cut diet plan. They break the monotony of eating the same types of foods, day after day, and give you treats to look forward to on the weekends. You can choose any food you'd like as a cheat meal as long as you choose small portions—about the size of your fist. That will keep your calories in the range to continue your weight loss.

Cheats break up the monotony day in, day out, and let you reward yourself—in a small way—after sticking to The Cut for a week. They also let you indulge in your favorite foods, and you learn how to include smaller portions of even unhealthy foods without overeating. That will help you maintain your fat loss even after you complete The Cut.

From Obi:

I usually go to the grocery store after I work out, so I'm there in a tank top and shorts, so people can tell I'm in shape. That's a double-edged sword—I'll see people checking out my shopping cart. I usually have chicken breasts and turkey breasts and healthy options in the basket, but I'll also have items like dried pineapple, popcorn, and chocolate chip cookies. I've always got to have the cheats, but sometimes I feel like I have to justify them when I check out. I even had a grocery store clerk call me out on my cookies and popcorn and tell me that stuff isn't healthy. That stuff is my cheat meal, and I have to indulge sometimes!

The Importance of Water

What's the absolute best beverage you can consume to help you lose weight, stay healthy, and have more energy? Water. The question is, how much do you need? Well, you get some water—about 20 percent of your daily intake—from the food you eat. Fruits and vegetables and other foods like soup have a high water content, so consuming them also satisfies some of your hydration needs.

The amount of water you need to function optimally will depend on your age, weight, activity level, and even environment. Aim to drink at least eight 8-ounce glasses of water every day for optimal hydration and digestion. Carry a water bottle so you drink before, during, and after your workout to prevent dehydration, especially if you tend to sweat a lot. Exercising while dehydrated can cause muscle cramps and fatigue, the last thing you want when you're working out!

THE BIG PICTURE

Now that you understand the *why* of the Cut diet, let's take the next step and get into the *how*. You'll find the Cut meal plans in the next chapter.

5 The Cut Meal Plans

Choosing the One That's Right for You

To get started on the Cut meal plan, choose the weight category that matches your current body weight. You'll find the plans for men listed first, and then the plans for women. Look at the following chart to determine your starting weight, and then turn to the pages that include your personalized Cut meal plan:

MEN:	
Starting Weight	*Starting Daily Caloric Intake*
220+ pounds	2,200 to 2,250 calories
180–219 pounds	2,000 to 2,050 calories
160–179 pounds	1,800 to 1,850 calories
Under 160 pounds	1,600 to 1,650 calories

WOMEN:	
Starting Weight	*Starting Daily Caloric Intake*
220+ pounds	1,700 to 1,750 calories
180–219 pounds	1,600 to 1,650 calories
160–179 pounds	1,500 to 1,550 calories
140–159 pounds	1,400 to 1,450 calories
Under 140 pounds	1,300 to 1,350 calories

Making the Cut: Real People, Real Results

Name: Dionne Davis

Age: 43

Location: Rock Hill, South Carolina

Occupation: CEO and founder, *FitFigures* magazine

Height: 5'8"

Starting weight: 198 pounds

Ending weight: 180 pounds

When I first started The Cut, I felt very full because I was actually eating food on a regular schedule, and tired because I wasn't used to going to the gym five days a week. After about two weeks, my body became a clock and knew when it was time to eat. Because I had the right nutrients in my body, I was ready for and looked forward to my workouts.

Going to the gym five days a week was a challenge but I quickly became a gym rat…and after just two weeks, I noticed a difference in my body. I took pictures every two or three weeks, so I could actually *see* a difference. Now I feel fantastic, and The Cut definitely curbed my sugar intake. I've learned how to eat to live, rather than live to eat.

> Now I feel fantastic, and The Cut definitely curbed my sugar intake. I've learned how to eat to live, rather than live to eat.

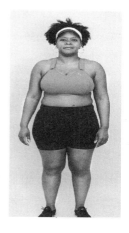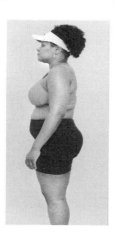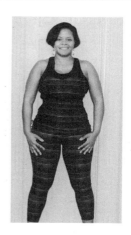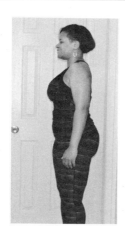

DAILY CALORIE TARGET CHART

You already know the number of calories you'll consume during the first four weeks of The Cut. You'll decrease the number of calories you consume during the next four weeks, and again the four weeks after that, to spur fat loss and avoid weight loss plateaus:

Initial (Weeks 1–4) Calorie Target	Weeks 5–8 Calorie Target	Weeks 9–12 Calorie Target
2,200	2,000	1,800
2,000	1,800	1,600
1,800	1,600	1,500
1,700	1,500	1,300
1,600	1,500	1,400
1,500	1,400	1,300
1,400	1,300	1,200
1,300	1,300*	1,200

At this calorie level, you'll consume 1,300 calories for the first eight weeks, and then drop to 1,200 for the last four weeks.

Protein Powder: A Valuable Addition to the Cut Plan

When you look at the Cut meal plans, you'll see that each day includes a protein drink. Your protein drink is a scoop of protein powder, mixed with water.

Look for a protein powder that's whey-based (it's digested more quickly than other proteins) and contains no more than 2 grams of sugar per serving. A typical protein powder will provide about 20 grams of protein for about 120 calories.

A Note About Fish Oil

In the Cut meal plans below, you'll see that we suggest you have a serving of fish oil (2 capsules) at breakfast. If you're already having a serving of healthy fat at breakfast, you can choose to skip the fish oil. We've included it as an option because most Americans don't consume enough of these heart-healthy fats—and one serving of fish oil will not in any way derail your weight loss plans!

THE CUT MEAL PLANS

Here are the Cut meal plans, based on calorie targets. Choose the one that you'll use for the first four weeks:

2,200-Calorie Cut Meal Plan

If your goal is 2,200 calories, each day you'll consume:

- 7 lean proteins
- 6 starchy carbs
- 5 fibrous carbs
- 6 healthy fats

You will have two servings of protein, two servings of starchy carbs, one to two servings of fibrous carbs, and one to two servings of healthy fats (depending on the meal) each meal, along with two servings of healthy fats as a midafternoon snack. Two days a week, you will swap out two meals (for four meals total) as cheat meals. (You can eat whatever you want for your cheat meals—as long as the portion is no larger than your fist.)

Here's the meal plan blueprint:

Morning (or before working out)

Protein shake (P)

Breakfast

P P
SC SC
C
F

Lunch

P P
SC SC
C C
F

Snack

F F

Dinner

P P

SC SC

C C

F F

Here's what a day on the plan might look like:

Morning (or before working out)

Protein shake (P)

Breakfast

2 eggs, cooked any way (2 P)

1 cup cooked oatmeal, plain (2 SC)

1 banana (C)

2 fish oil capsules (F)

Lunch

6 ounces chicken breast, chopped (2 P)

1 cup black beans (2 SC)

4 cups spinach-and-kale mix (2 C)

2 teaspoons olive oil (F)

Snack

¼ cup unsalted almonds (about 24 almonds) (2 F)

Dinner

Carne Asada Tacos (2 servings) (see recipe, page 102) (2 P 2 SC 2 F)

2 cups steamed broccoli or mixed vegetables (2 C)

> *Here's what another day on the plan might look like:*

Morning (or before working out)

Protein shake (P)

Breakfast

Huevos Rancheros (make with an extra egg) (see recipe, page 91) (2 P SC C F)
½ cup cooked oatmeal, plain (SC)
2 fish oil capsules (F) (optional)

Lunch

Creole Kidney Beans (2 servings) (see recipe, page 98) (2 P 2 SC 2 C 2 F)

Snack

2 tablespoons unsalted walnuts (about 12 walnut halves) (F)

Dinner

Buffalo Wings (2 servings) (see recipe, page 104) (2 P 2 F)
1 cup cooked brown rice (2 SC)
2 cups Simple Steamed Cauliflower (see recipe, page 97) (2 C)

2,000-Calorie Cut Meal Plan

If your goal is 2,000 calories, each day you'll consume:

- 6 lean proteins
- 5 starchy carbs
- 5 fibrous carbs
- 6 healthy fats

You will have one to two servings of protein, one to two servings of starchy carbs, one to two servings of fibrous carbs, and one serving of healthy fats at each meal, and a midafternoon snack of two servings of healthy fats. Two days a week, you will swap out two meals (for four meals total) as cheat meals. (You can eat whatever you want for your cheat meals—as long as the portion is no larger than your fist.)

Here's the meal plan blueprint:

Morning (or before working out)

Protein shake (P)

Breakfast

P
SC SC
C
F

Lunch

P P
SC SC
C C
F

Snack

F F

Dinner

P P
SC
C C
F F

Here's what a day on the plan might look like:

Morning (or before working out)

Protein shake (P)

Breakfast

1 egg, scrambled or hard-boiled (P)
1 cup cooked oatmeal, plain (2 SC)
1 cup strawberries (C)
2 fish oil capsules (F)

Lunch

Creole Kidney Beans (2 servings) (see recipe, page 98) (2 P 2 SC 2 C 2 F)

Snack

2 tablespoons unsalted almonds (about 12 almonds) (F)

Dinner

Baked Salmon and Asparagus Bundles (2 servings) (see recipe, page 109) (2 P 2 C 2 F)
1 small baked potato, plain (SC)

Here's what another day on the plan might look like:

Morning (or before working out)

Protein shake (P)

Breakfast

Huevos Rancheros (see recipe, page 91) (P SC C F)
2 fish oil capsules (F) (optional)

Lunch

Warm Chard, Kale, and White Bean Salad (2 servings) (see recipe, page 95) (2 P 2 SC 2 C 2 F)

Snack

2 tablespoons unsalted pistachios (about 24) (F)

Dinner

Steak Barcelona (2 servings) (see recipe, page 107) (2 P 2 C 2 F)

½ cup cooked brown rice (SC)

Here's what another day on the plan might look like:

Morning (or before working out)

Protein shake (P)

Breakfast

Southwestern Tofu Scramble (2 servings) (see recipe, page 91) (2 P 2 SC 2 C 2 F)

2 fish oil capsules (F) (optional)

Lunch

6 ounces cooked chicken or turkey breast, chopped, for salad (2 P)

2 cups mixed salad greens with 1 cup chopped carrots and peppers, and 1 cup white beans (2 C 2 SC)

2 teaspoons olive oil (to top salad)(F)

Snack

¼ cup unsalted almonds (about 24 almonds) (2 F)

Dinner

Simple Oven-Roasted Chicken Breast (2 servings) (see recipe, page 101) (2 P 2 F)

1 small baked potato, plain (SC)

2 cups Simple Steamed Broccoli (see recipe, page 97) (2 C)

1,800-Calorie Cut Meal Plan

If your goal is 1,800 calories, each day you'll consume:

- 5 lean proteins
- 5 starchy carbs
- 5 fibrous carbs
- 5 healthy fats

You will have one to two servings of protein, one to two servings of starchy carbs, one to two servings of fibrous carbs, and one healthy serving of healthy fats each meal; you'll also have two servings of healthy fats as a midafternoon snack. Two days a week, you will swap out two meals (for four meals total) as cheat meals. (You can eat whatever you want for your cheat meals—as long as the portion is no larger than your fist.)

Here's the meal plan blueprint:

Morning (or before working out)

Protein shake (P)

Breakfast

P
SC
C
F

Lunch

P P
SC SC
C C
F

Snack

F F

Dinner

P
SC SC
C C
F

Here's what a day on the plan might look like:

Morning (or before working out)

Protein shake (P)

Breakfast

Southwestern Tofu Scramble (see recipe, page 91) (P SC C F)

2 fish oil capsules (F) (optional)

Lunch

6 ounces chicken breast, chopped (to top spinach) (2 P)

2 cups spinach topped with 1 cup chopped carrots and bell peppers and 1 cup white beans (2 C 2 SC)

2 teaspoons olive oil (F)

Snack

¼ cup unsalted almonds (about 24 almonds) (2 F)

Dinner

Crispy Baked Fish and Kale (see recipe, page 108) (P C F)

1 cup quinoa, prepared per package directions (2 SC)

Here's what another day on the plan might look like:

Morning (or before working out)

Protein shake (P)

Breakfast

1 egg, hard-boiled (P)

½ cup cooked oatmeal, plain (SC)

1 cup strawberries (add to oatmeal) (C)

2 fish oil capsules (F)

Lunch

Buffalo Turkey Lettuce Wraps (2 servings) (see recipe, page 110) (2 P 2 C 2 F)
1 cup cooked brown rice (2 SC)

Snack

2 tablespoons unsalted walnuts (about 12 walnut halves) (F)

Dinner

Apple-Dijon Pork Chop (see recipe, page 104) (P C F)
1 cup millet, cooked according to package directions (2 SC)

1,700-Calorie Cut Meal Plan

If your goal is 1,700 calories, each day you'll consume:

- 5 lean proteins
- 4 starchy carbs
- 5 fibrous carbs
- 4 healthy fats

You will have one to two servings of protein, one to two servings of starchy carbs, one to two servings of fibrous carbs, and one to two servings of healthy fats each meal; you'll also have one serving of fibrous carbs as a midafternoon snack. Two days a week, you will swap out two meals (for four meals total) as cheat meals. (You can eat whatever you want for your cheat meals—as long as the portion is no larger than your fist.)

Here's the meal plan blueprint:

Morning (or before working out)

Protein shake (P)

Breakfast

P
SC SC
C
F

Lunch

 P
 SC
 C
 F

Snack

 C

Dinner

 P P
 SC
 C C
 F F

Here's what a day on the plan might look like:

Morning (or before working out)

 Protein shake (P)

Breakfast

 1 cup nonfat Greek yogurt (P)
 1 cup cooked oatmeal, plain (2 SC)
 1 cup strawberries (C)
 2 fish oil capsules (F)

Lunch

 Warm Chard, Kale, and White Bean Salad (see recipe, page 95) (P SC C F)

Snack

 1 small apple (C)

Dinner

Jerk Shrimp with Lime-Infused Pineapple (2 servings) (see recipe, page 108) (2 P 2 C 2 F)

½ cup quinoa, prepared per package directions (SC)

Here's what another day on the plan might look like:

Morning (or before working out)

Protein shake (P)

Breakfast

Huevos Rancheros (see recipe, page 91) (P SC C F)

2 fish oil capsules (F) (optional)

½ cup cooked oatmeal, plain (SC)

Lunch

Moroccan Bean Salad (see recipe, page 96) (P SC C F)

Snack

1 small banana (C)

Dinner

Baked Salmon and Asparagus Bundles (2 servings) (see recipe, page 109) (2 P 2 C 2 F)

½ cup cooked brown rice (SC)

1,600-Calorie Cut Meal Plan

If your goal is 1,600 calories, each day you'll consume:

- 5 lean proteins
- 3 starchy carbs
- 5 fibrous carbs
- 4 healthy fats

You will have one to two servings of protein, one serving of starchy carbs, one to two servings of fibrous carbs, and one to two servings of healthy fats each meal; you'll also have one serving of fibrous carbs as a midafternoon snack. Two days a week, you will swap out two meals (for four meals total) as cheat meals. (You can eat whatever you want for your cheat meals—as long as the portion is no larger than your fist.)

Here's the meal plan blueprint:

Morning (or before working out)

Protein shake (P)

Breakfast

P
SC
C
F

Lunch

P
SC
C
F F

Snack

C

Dinner

P P
SC
C C
F

Here's what a day on the plan might look like:

Morning (or before working out)

Protein shake (P)

Breakfast

Huevos Rancheros (see recipe, page 91) (P SC C F)
2 fish oil capsules (F) (optional)

Lunch

Beef Noodle Pho (see recipe, page 111) (P SC C F)

Snack

1 medium apple (C)

Dinner

Baked Salmon and Asparagus Bundles (2 servings) (see recipe, page 109)
(2 P 2 C 2 F)
½ cup quinoa, prepared per package directions (SC)

Here's what another day on the plan might look like:

Morning (or before working out)

Protein shake (P)

Breakfast

Southwestern Tofu Scramble (see recipe, page 91) (P SC C F)
2 fish oil capsules (F) (optional)

Lunch

Simple Oven-Roasted Chicken Breast, chopped (see recipe, page 101) (P F)
½ cup cooked brown rice (SC)
2 cups mixed greens topped with 2 teaspoons olive oil (C F)

Snack

2 small plums (C)

Dinner

Apple-Dijon Pork Chop (with an extra serving of pork) (see recipe, page 104) (2 P C F)

1 small baked potato, plain (SC)

1 cup Simple Steamed Carrots (see recipe, page 97) (C)

1,500-Calorie Cut Meal Plan

If your goal is 1,500 calories, each day you'll consume:

- 4 lean proteins
- 3 starchy carbs
- 5 fibrous carbs
- 4 healthy fats

You will have one serving of protein, one serving of starchy carbs, one to two servings of fibrous carbs, and one to two servings of healthy fats each meal; you'll also have one serving of fibrous carbs as a midafternoon snack. Two days a week, you will swap out two meals (for four meals total) as cheat meals. (You can eat whatever you want for your cheat meals—as long as the portion is no larger than your fist.)

Here's the meal plan blueprint:

Morning (or before working out)

Protein shake (P)

Breakfast

P

SC

C C

F

Lunch

 P

 SC

 C

 F

Snack

 C

Dinner

 P

 SC

 C

 F F

Here's what a day on the plan might look like:

Morning (or before working out)

Protein shake (P)

Breakfast

Loaded Breakfast Potato Skins (see recipe, page 92) (P SC F)

2 fish oil capsules (F) (optional)

1 orange (C)

Lunch

Classic Greek Salad (see recipe, page 96) (P C F)

½ cup white beans (add to salad) (SC)

Snack

1 medium apple (C)

Dinner

Jerk Shrimp with Lime-Infused Pineapple (see recipe, page 108) (P C F)
½ cup cooked brown rice (SC)

Here's what another day on the plan might look like:

Morning (or before working out)

Protein shake (P)

Breakfast

1 egg, scrambled (P)
½ cup cooked oatmeal, plain (SC)
2 cups strawberries (2 C)
2 fish oil capsules (F)

Lunch

Beef Noodle Pho (see recipe, page 111) (P SC C F)·

Snack

2 small plums (C) and 2 tablespoons unsalted walnuts (F)

Dinner

Steak Barcelona (see recipe, page 107) (P C F)
½ cup cooked brown rice (SC)

1,400-Calorie Cut Meal Plan

If your goal is 1,400 calories, each day you'll consume:

- 4 lean proteins
- 3 starchy carbs
- 5 fibrous carbs
- 3 healthy fats

You will have one serving of protein, one serving of starchy carbs, one to two servings of fibrous carbs, and one serving of healthy fats each meal; you'll also have one serving of fibrous carbs as a midafternoon snack. Two days a week, you will swap out two meals (for four meals total) as cheat meals. (You can eat whatever you want for your cheat meals—as long as the portion is no larger than your fist.)

Here's the meal plan blueprint:

Morning (or before working out)

Protein shake (P)

Breakfast

P
SC
C
F

Lunch

P
SC
C
F

Snack

C

Dinner

P
SC
C C
F

Here's what a day on the plan might look like:

Morning (or before working out)

Protein shake (P)

Breakfast

Southwestern Tofu Scramble (see recipe, page 91) (P SC C F)
2 fish oil capsules (F) (optional)

Lunch

Buffalo Turkey Lettuce Wraps (see recipe, page 110) (P C F)
½ cup cooked brown rice (SC)

Snack

2 small tangerines (C)

Dinner

Grilled Greek Yogurt Chicken (see recipe, page 105) (P C F)
½ cup quinoa, prepared per package directions (SC)
1 cup Simple Steamed Spinach (see recipe, page 97) (C)

Here's what another day on the plan might look like:

Morning (or before working out)

Protein shake (P)

Breakfast

1 cup plain nonfat yogurt (P)
½ cup cooked oatmeal, plain (SC)
1 cup cantaloupe, cut into pieces (C)
2 fish oil capsules (F)

Lunch

Creole Kidney Beans (see recipe, page 98) (P SC C F)

Snack

1 apple (C)

Dinner

Roasted Garlic Spaghetti Squash "Ramen" (see recipe, page 94) (P C F)
½ cup cooked brown rice (SC)
1 cup Simple Steamed Green Beans (see recipe, page 97) (C)

1,300-Calorie Cut Meal Plan

If your goal is 1,300 calories, each day you'll consume:

- 4 lean proteins
- 3 starchy carbs
- 4 fibrous carbs
- 3 healthy fats

You will have one serving of protein, one serving of starchy carbs, one serving of fibrous carbs, and one serving of healthy fats each meal; you'll also have one serving of fibrous carbs as a midafternoon snack. Two days a week, you will swap out two meals (for four meals total) as cheat meals. (You can eat whatever you want for your cheat meals—as long as the portion is no larger than your fist.)

Here's the meal plan blueprint:

Morning (or before working out)

Protein shake (P)

Breakfast

P
SC
C
F

Lunch

P

SC

C

F

Snack

C

Dinner

P

SC

C

F

Here's what a day on the plan might look like:

Morning (or before working out)

Protein shake (P)

Breakfast

1 cup nonfat Greek yogurt (P)

½ cup cooked oatmeal, plain (SC)

1 cup strawberries (C)

2 fish oil capsules (F)

Lunch

Pesto Chicken Soup (see recipe, page 93) (P C F)

½ cup white beans (add to soup) (SC)

Snack

2 small plums (C)

Dinner

Steak Barcelona (see recipe, page 107) (P C F)

½ cup cooked brown rice (SC)

Here's what another day on the plan might look like:

Morning (or before working out)

Protein shake (P)

Breakfast

Homemade Granola (see recipe, page 90) (P SC C F)

Lunch

Moroccan Bean Salad (see recipe, page 96) (P SC C F)

Snack

1 medium apple (C)

Dinner

Baked Salmon and Asparagus Bundles (see recipe, page 109) (P C F)

½ cup whole-grain pasta (SC)

1,200-Calorie Cut Meal Plan

If your goal is 1,200 calories, each day you'll consume:

- 4 lean proteins
- 2 starchy carbs
- 4 fibrous carbs
- 3 healthy fats

You will have one serving of protein, one serving of starchy carbs, one serving of fibrous carbs, and one serving of healthy fats two meals a day; for the third meal, you'll have one serving of protein, fibrous carbs, and healthy fat. You'll also have an afternoon snack of fibrous carbs. Two days a week, you will swap out two meals (for four meals total) as cheat meals. (You can eat whatever you want for your cheat meals—as long as the portion is no larger than your fist.)

Here's the meal plan blueprint:

Morning (or before working out)

Protein shake (P)

Breakfast

P
SC
C
F

Lunch

P
SC
C
F

Snack

C

Dinner

P
C
F

Here's what a day on the plan might look like:

Morning (or before working out)

Protein shake (P)

Breakfast

1 egg, hard-boiled (P)

½ cup cooked oatmeal, plain (SC)

1 cup blueberries (C)

2 fish oil capsules (F)

Lunch

Simple Oven-Roasted Chicken Breast (see recipe, page 101) (P F)

½ cup cooked brown rice (SC)

1 cup Simple Steamed Green Beans (see recipe, page 97) (C)

Snack

1 medium apple (C)

Dinner

Crispy Baked Fish and Kale (see recipe, page 108) (P C F)

Here's what another day on the plan might look like:

Morning (or before working out)

Protein shake (P)

Breakfast

Huevos Rancheros (see recipe, page 91) (P SC C F)

2 fish oil capsules (F) (optional)

Lunch

Warm Chard, Kale, and White Bean Salad (see recipe, page 95) (P SC C F)

Snack

1 orange (C)

Dinner

Apple-Dijon Pork Chop (see recipe, page 104) (P C F)

From Obi:

Feeling hungry between meals and don't want to blow your diet? Vegetables are your best low-calorie snack. They're high in fiber, which helps suppress your appetite, and loaded with nutrients you need. A handful of baby carrots, sliced peppers, or even raw broccoli can satisfy an urge to crunch and take the edge off your appetite so you don't overeat at dinner.

Making the Cut: Real People, Real Results

Name: Sharad Cara
Age: 51
Location: Cape Town, South Africa
Occupation: Orthodontist
Height: 5'9"
Starting weight: 202.8 pounds
Ending weight: 182.5 pounds

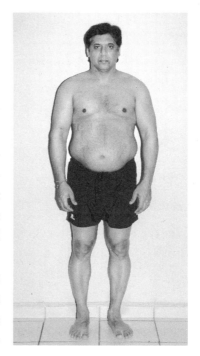

Over the last 20 years, I've tried at least six different diet and exercise plans and worked with personal trainers, but haven't been able to lose weight and keep it off. One of the things I liked about The Cut was that it offered structure for both the meal plan and the training plan.

I would love to do the weights and cardio in one session, but I just don't have enough time in the mornings. So I did the weight training in the morning, before work, and the cardio in the evening, after work.

This whole program has been life changing for me. My daily routine has changed. My training routine has improved. My eating habits have changed. I am feeling so much fitter and stronger. My resting pulse rate has dropped from an average of 69 to 59.

When I wake up in the morning, it is so noticeably easy for me to sit up in bed—because I have been doing so many sit-ups in this program. The simple act of putting on my socks and tying my shoelaces is effortless.

My success on The Cut has affected my family as well. My wife realized that she can cook the Cut foods, so my family now eats the same healthy dinners together. My wife and kids have seen the difference in my body, and they know that my diet played a huge role, so they want to eat like me!

In 12 weeks, I lost 5 inches around my waist and lowered my body fat percentage by 5 percent on the program. That's incredible! I know that this way of life will stay with me forever and it has definitely inspired my family. I can *highly* recommend this program to anyone. I have firsthand experience that it definitely works.

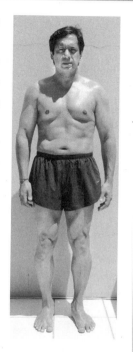

In 12 weeks, I lost 5 inches around my waist and lowered my body fat percentage by 5 percent on the program. That's incredible!

From Obi:

Don't blame your slow metabolism for being overweight—blame bad lifestyle choices! Living healthfully is a lifestyle, folks!

From Obi: Morris's Cut Diet Plan

I designed the following meal plan for Morris, and it helped him lose 33 pounds in just 12 weeks. I tweaked the plan a bit and had him consume a midmorning protein snack and a post-workout protein shake (in addition to a pre-workout shake) to help him build as much muscle and shed as much fat as possible. Morris thrives on consistency, so he ate the same meals for weeks on end. (He did swap in turkey, chicken, and lean beef for proteins, but his basic meals stayed the same.) But when you do The Cut, you'll have plenty of options to swap in and out to ensure a variety of delicious meals that will burn off your excess body fat.

Morris started out on the 2,200-calorie-a-day plan for the first four weeks on The Cut. His calorie goal dropped to 2,000 per day the next four weeks, and 1,800 calories a day the last four weeks, resulting in his phenomenal weight loss.

Curious about what his actual meal plan looked like? Here's what he ate during the first four weeks and the food group breakdown:

Morning
    1 scoop whey protein mixed with water before working out and 1 scoop
        whey protein mixed with water immediately after working out (2 P)

Breakfast
    5 egg whites (P)
    1 cup cooked oatmeal with 2 teaspoons brown sugar (2 SC)
    1 banana (C)
    2 fish oil capsules (F)

Midmorning Snack
    3 ounces water-packed white tuna, eaten plain (P)

Lunch
    6 ounces baked or broiled chicken breast, cooked with 2 teaspoons olive oil
        (2 P 2 F)
    1 cup cooked brown rice (2 SC)
    2 cups cooked spinach (2 C)

Midafternoon Snack

½ cup unsalted almonds (4 F)*

Dinner

6 ounces baked turkey breast (2 P)

2 small baked potatoes, plain (2 SC)

2 cups cooked broccoli (2 C)

*Note: Morris chose to have more healthy fats for his midafternoon snack instead of having some with his dinner, and had several extra servings of protein to add as much muscle as possible. He was extraordinarily committed to staying on The Cut, but I suggest you always have a healthy fat at dinner to help you feel full and satisfied longer.

And in case you're wondering, yes, Morris did enjoy cheats on the weekends—his favorite cheat is a (small) serving of dessert.

6 The Cut Recipes

Delicious, Simple Meals to Help You Shed Fat

In the last two chapters, you learned the basics of the Cut meal plans. This chapter gives you simple recipes that are based on Cut principles. If you're someone who always relies on fast food or prepackaged food, we encourage you to spend some time in the kitchen! Cooking your own food lets you control what goes into it (and what doesn't) and will save you money in the long run, too.

Sure, Morris ate the same thing day after day when he followed the Cut plan, but we know most people need more variety in their diet to stick to it! We also know that you may not be an experienced cook, so you'll find some super-simple one-ingredient recipes (like how to cook a chicken breast or steam fresh vegetables). Then you'll find more complex (but still simple) ones that contain several of the types of foods you should be eating on The Cut. Feel free to swap different foods in the recipes (for example, white-fish instead of salmon) as you like.

Best part? These healthy recipes are ones that you can make part of your regular routine even after you finish the Cut program.

Each recipe:

- Is simple to prepare;
- Is delicious;
- Is based on healthy foods your body needs; and
- Contains fewer than 500 calories.

About the Cut Recipes

You now have the building blocks for how to eat on the Cut plan. The recipes in this chapter are meant to give you greater variety and to show you that you can enjoy delicious meals—while sticking to the Cut principles. You may notice that while each recipe contains the foods you should be basing your diet on for life, some do contain small amounts of ingredients (such as bacon or cheese) that aren't part of the Cut plan. Some of the recipes include slightly larger servings of protein (4 ounces versus 3 ounces) as well. Don't worry about that—we've accounted for the difference in calories, and these recipes are designed for success on the Cut plan.

Making the Recipes Part of Your Cut Plan

We've made it simple for you to include these recipes as part of The Cut by telling you what macronutrients (protein, starchy carbs, fibrous carbs, and healthy fats) each serving includes. You'll find the key at the end of each recipe to make it easy for you to incorporate these delicious dishes into your diet.

BREAKFAST RECIPES

Homemade Granola

Serves 2

Sure, you can buy granola, but it may be loaded with sugar and other ingredients you don't want. Why not make a healthier version yourself? You'll minimize the sugar and fat, and maximize the nutrients and flavor.

INGREDIENTS

¼ cup rolled oats

2 teaspoons sesame seeds

2 teaspoons sunflower seeds

2 teaspoons flaxseeds

¼ cup chopped pecans

Pinch of sea salt

2 teaspoons coconut oil

2 teaspoons honey

2 tablespoons raisins

2 tablespoons dried cranberries

½ cup nonfat milk

METHOD

1. Preheat the oven to 350°F. Place parchment paper on a baking sheet. In a large bowl combine the oats, sesame seeds, sunflower seeds, flaxseeds, pecans, and salt. Combine the coconut oil and honey in a microwavable container and warm for 10 seconds, then stir into the bowl.

2. Spread the mixture out onto the prepared baking sheet in a thin layer. Bake for 30 minutes until well toasted, stirring every 5 minutes to ensure even baking. Let it cool completely, then mix in the dried fruit.

3. Serve with the nonfat milk.

383 calories per serving. Store in an airtight container if you don't eat right away. Each serving: P, SC, C, F.

Huevos Rancheros

Nothing gets you moving in the morning like savory south-of-the-border flavors.

INGREDIENTS

2 teaspoons olive oil

2 scallions, chopped

2 cloves garlic, minced

2 medium tomatoes, diced

½ cup black beans, drained and rinsed

2 large eggs, whisked

2 wheat-flour tortillas

2 tablespoons salsa

2 tablespoons plain nonfat yogurt

½ avocado, diced (½ cup)

2 tablespoons cilantro leaves, chopped

METHOD

1. Heat the oil in a large skillet over medium-high heat. Add the scallions and garlic; cook until tender. Add the tomatoes and beans. Cook to warm through and reduce any liquid. Add the eggs and stir continuously until cooked. Remove from the heat.

2. Warm the tortillas by brushing lightly over a stovetop burner, or in the microwave for 10 seconds. Place each tortilla on a plate, then top with the egg mixture, salsa, yogurt, avocado, and cilantro. Serve immediately.

402 calories per serving. Each serving: P, SC, C, F.

Southwestern Tofu Scramble

Tofu lovers know that the beauty of this ingredient is its ability to absorb flavors. This version has mild spices, but you can increase the heat as much as you dare. Even meat eaters will love this dish!

(continued)

INGREDIENTS

8 ounces firm tofu

2 teaspoons olive oil

½ cup diced red onion

2 tablespoons diced red bell pepper

2 tablespoons diced jalapeño

2 cloves garlic, minced

½ teaspoon cumin

½ teaspoon coriander

½ teaspoon chili powder

½ cup corn kernels (canned or frozen)

½ cup black beans, drained and rinsed

2 cups chopped kale

½ cup chopped cilantro

Pinch of sea salt and black pepper

METHOD

1. Place the unwrapped tofu on a plate, top with a second plate, and set aside to compress for 10 minutes. (This removes excess moisture, makes the tofu easier to slice, and helps it crumble into nice firm bits.)

2. Meanwhile, heat the oil in a large skillet over medium-high heat. Add the onion, bell pepper, jalapeño, and garlic; cook until tender. Add the spices, corn, and beans, and cook to warm through. Crumble the tofu and add it to the pan. Cook while stirring to thoroughly blend the flavors. Finish by adding the kale and cilantro. Cook, stirring, until the kale is wilted. Season with salt and pepper and serve immediately.

272 calories per serving. Each serving: P, SC, C, F.

Loaded Breakfast Potato Skins

Serves 2

This recipe puts a new twist on standard breakfast fare. It's at home at brunch or during halftime of the big game.

INGREDIENTS

2 small russet potatoes (about 2 inches in diameter), baked in oven or microwave

2 slices bacon, diced

2 large eggs, beaten

Pinch of sea salt and black pepper

¼ cup grated cheddar cheese

2 tablespoons nonfat yogurt

2 tablespoons chopped chives or scallions

METHOD

1. Preheat the oven to 375°F. Place parchment paper on a baking sheet. Slice the already-baked potato into quarters lengthwise. Scoop out most of the white inner potato, leaving just ½ inch clinging to the skin. Set skin-side down on a baking sheet. (Save the inner potato for use in another recipe.)

2. Cook the bacon in a small skillet over medium heat until the fat is rendered and the meat is crispy. Drain off all but 1 teaspoon of the fat. Add the beaten eggs, salt, and pepper; cook, stirring, until firm. Divide the egg evenly onto the top of each skin. Top each skin with cheddar cheese. Bake for 5 to 10 minutes, until the cheese is melted and bubbly. Serve topped with yogurt and chopped chives.

377 calories per serving. Each serving: P, SC, F.

SOUPS/SALADS/SIDE DISHES

Pesto Chicken Soup

Serves 2

This recipe is the perfect way to use up your leftover grilled, broiled, or poached chicken. When you're cooking chicken throughout the week, make a little extra to keep on hand. You can swap in turkey or even canned chicken in a pinch.

INGREDIENTS

2 teaspoons olive oil

½ cup diced yellow onion

2 stalks celery, chopped

½ cup diced carrot

4 cloves garlic, minced

4 cups basil, chopped

2 cups chopped or shredded cooked chicken

2 cups chicken broth

Pinch of sea salt and black pepper

2 tablespoons store-bought pesto

(continued)

METHOD

1. Heat the oil in a large skillet over medium heat. Add the onion, celery, and carrot; cook until tender and just beginning to caramelize or turn brown. Add the garlic, basil, and chicken meat. Cook, stirring, to warm through, about 3 to 5 minutes.

2. Slowly add the broth, salt, and pepper. Bring just to a boil. Season with salt and pepper as needed, then transfer to a soup bowl. Garnish with the pesto and serve.

306 calories per serving. Can be kept in the refrigerator for up to a week before eating. Each serving: P, C, F.

Roasted Garlic Spaghetti Squash "Ramen"

Serves 2

Spaghetti squash is magical. It's great on its own, but it's even more fun when standing in for higher-calorie pasta. Here, the added sweetness really rounds out the ramen broth flavors.

INGREDIENTS

2 spaghetti squash

1 teaspoon toasted sesame oil

2 cloves garlic, minced

2 teaspoons freshly grated gingerroot

6 large shiitake or button mushrooms

2 cups vegetable or chicken broth, warmed

2 tablespoons soy sauce

3 cups baby spinach, chopped

2 scallions, chopped

2 hard-boiled eggs, chopped into pieces

METHOD

1. Preheat the oven to 375°F. Cut each spaghetti squash in half lengthwise. Scoop out the seeds, and place the hollowed halves on a baking sheet with a rim, cut-side down. Add ¼ inch of water to the pan and bake until tender, about 30 to 45 minutes. Let the squash cool.

2. Meanwhile, heat the sesame oil in a large sauté pan over medium-high heat. Add the garlic, ginger, and mushrooms, and stir until fragrant and just browned. Reduce the heat and carefully add the broth and soy sauce. Set aside to simmer over low heat until the squash is done baking.

3. Gently scrape out the interior of the squash from its skin with a fork. It will shred on its own into spaghetti-like strands (hence the name). Place 1 cup of the strands in a large soup bowl. (Store the rest in the fridge or freezer for future recipes. It's great served with just a little salt and olive oil.)

4. Place the spinach and scallions on top of the squash. Bring the broth to a boil and immediately pour it into the bowl. (You can pour it through a strainer if you'd like to remove the garlic and ginger bits.) Top with the eggs. Serve immediately!

262 calories per serving. Each serving: P, C, F.

Warm Chard, Kale, and White Bean Salad

Serves 2

Warm salads are a crunchy alternative to standard vegetable side dishes. But with the added protein from the beans, this recipe is a meal in itself.

INGREDIENTS

2 teaspoons olive oil

2 cloves garlic, minced

½ cup chopped red onion

2 teaspoons dried thyme

Grated zest and juice of 2 oranges

½ teaspoon sea salt

1 cup white beans, drained and rinsed

2 cups Swiss chard, rinsed and chopped

2 cups kale, rinsed and chopped

METHOD

Heat the oil in a large skillet over medium heat. Add the garlic, onion, and thyme, and cook, stirring, until onion has softened, about 1 minute. Add the orange zest, juice, and salt; warm through for another minute. Add the beans and toss to coat. Add the chard and kale, and toss until well coated, then remove from the heat. Serve.

383 calories per serving. Store in an airtight container if you don't eat immediately. Each serving: P, SC, C, F.

Moroccan Bean Salad

Serves 2

The spice blend in this recipe is an exotic departure from the standard bland bean salad.

INGREDIENTS

2 small cloves garlic, minced

2 tablespoons chopped mint leaves

1 teaspoon sea salt

2 teaspoons sesame seeds

½ teaspoon cumin

¼ teaspoon cinnamon

2 tablespoons olive oil

2 tablespoons lemon juice

1 cup garbanzo beans, drained and rinsed

1 cup white or kidney beans, drained and rinsed

½ cup grated carrot

½ cup parsley leaves

2 tablespoons prepared harissa, or prepared hot pepper chili paste

METHOD

In a large bowl, combine the garlic, mint, salt, sesame, cumin, and cinnamon. Stir together, crushing the ingredients to thoroughly combine the flavors. Slowly stir in the oil, then the lemon juice. Add the garbanzo and kidney beans, carrot, and parsley; toss well to coat everything. Serve topped with a dollop of harissa (to taste).

418 calories per serving. Store in an airtight container if you don't eat immediately. Each serving: P, SC, C, F.

Classic Greek Salad

Serves 2

This classic salad is too good to relegate to a side dish. Make it a hearty lunch or dinner, and let its Mediterranean flavors transport you to the Aegean.

INGREDIENTS

1 clove garlic	2 tablespoons olive oil
2 tablespoons fresh oregano	½ small red onion, sliced
Pinch of sea salt	½ cup diced tomato
6 kalamata olives, chopped	2 cups diced cucumber
Pinch of black pepper	½ cup Italian parsley leaves
2 teaspoons red wine vinegar	1 cup crumbled feta cheese

METHOD

Combine the garlic, oregano, and salt on a cutting board and mince them all together, creating a garlicky paste. Place this paste in a large bowl. Add the olives, pepper, vinegar, and oil; mix together. Add the onion, tomato, cucumber, and parsley, and toss to coat. Toss in the feta last. Serve chilled.

451 calories per serving. Store in an airtight container if you don't eat immediately. Each serving: P, C, F.

Simple Steamed Vegetables

Serves 2

Steaming vegetables cooks them while retaining their flavor and color and without losing nutrients. Cooking times will vary: asparagus takes 5 to 8 minutes; broccoli, 5 to 7 minutes; carrots, 10 to 15 minutes; cauliflower florets, 5 minutes; green beans, 4 to 6 minutes; and spinach and other greens, 2 to 3 minutes.

INGREDIENTS

4 cups fresh broccoli (or vegetable of your choice), chopped into equal-size pieces	Sea Salt
	Black Pepper

METHOD

1. Place a vegetable steamer in a medium- to large-size pot, add an inch or two of water, and bring the water to boil.
2. Add the broccoli to the steamer and cover; steam for 5 to 7 minutes, until cooked.
3. Season with a pinch of salt and/or pepper to taste. Serve.

110 calories per serving for broccoli. Store in an airtight container if you don't eat immediately. Each serving: 2 C.

Creole Kidney Beans

Serves 2

This vegetarian, protein-packed dish is delicious served with brown rice.

INGREDIENTS

1 red bell pepper, diced

1 green bell pepper, diced

2 stalks celery, diced

1 medium red onion, diced

1 tablespoon olive oil

½ teaspoon celery salt

½ teaspoon onion powder

½ teaspoon paprika

¼ teaspoon cayenne pepper (or to taste)

½ teaspoon dried thyme

¼ teaspoon dried basil

2 cloves garlic, minced

1 15-ounce can fire-roasted tomatoes (or regular diced tomatoes)

2 cups canned kidney beans, drained and rinsed

2 tablespoons chopped fresh parsley (optional)

METHOD

1. In a large sauté pan, sauté the peppers, celery, and onion in the olive oil for 5 to 7 minutes, until tender.

2. Add the celery salt, onion powder, paprika, cayenne, thyme, basil, and garlic. Sauté for 2 to 3 minutes until well blended. Add the tomatoes and kidney beans, and simmer uncovered for 8 to 10 minutes.

3. Serve, garnished with parsley if desired.

305 calories per serving. Store in an airtight container if you don't eat immediately. Each serving: P, SC, C, F.

Ginger, Spinach, and Mushroom Stir-Fry

Serves 2

This simple veggie side dish is the perfect complement to a lean protein and starchy carb.

INGREDIENTS

1 tablespoon balsamic vinegar

1 teaspoon ground ginger

1 teaspoon soy sauce

½ teaspoon garlic powder

2 cups mushrooms, sliced or quartered

1 tablespoon canola oil

4 cups raw spinach, washed

1 tablespoon unsalted sunflower seeds

METHOD

1. In a medium bowl, blend the vinegar, ginger, soy sauce, and garlic powder. Add the mushrooms and marinate for 5 minutes.
2. In a medium sauté pan over high heat, sauté the mushrooms in the canola oil until lightly brown. Add the spinach and cook for 1 to 2 minutes until just wilted, stirring constantly. Garnish with sunflower seeds and serve immediately.

160 calories per serving. Each serving: 2 C, F.

Oven-Roasted Sesame Orange Broccoli Florets

Serves 2

Roasting vegetables brings out their sweetness. This tasty dish will have you looking forward to getting your greens in.

INGREDIENTS

1 tablespoon canola oil

1 teaspoon soy sauce

1 teaspoon toasted sesame oil

1 teaspoon garlic powder

½ teaspoon black pepper

1 egg white

3 cups broccoli florets

2 tablespoons sesame seeds

2 oranges, peeled and cubed

(continued)

METHOD

1. Preheat the oven to 375°F and cover a baking sheet with parchment paper.
2. In a small bowl, blend the canola oil, soy sauce, sesame oil, spices, and egg white. Toss the broccoli in the mixture and spread evenly on the baking sheet. Sprinkle with the sesame seeds. Roast for 10 to 12 minutes until slightly browned on the edges. Toss the orange segments onto the baking sheet and bake for an additional 5 minutes, until the oranges are heated through. Serve immediately.

158 calories per serving. Each serving: 2 C, F.

Simple Salad

Serves 2

This simple recipe meets the requirements for the most basic Cut meal, with one serving of healthy protein, one serving of starchy carbs, one serving of fibrous carbs, and one serving of healthy fat. You can double the amounts of different foods to meet the requirements for that particular meal.

INGREDIENTS

4 cups mixed greens (or swap in any leafy greens)

1 cup white beans, drained and rinsed (or swap in any bean or legume)

3 ounces cooked chicken breast, chopped or shredded (or swap in any protein)

2 teaspoons olive oil (or swap in 1 teaspoon sunflower seeds or chopped nuts)

METHOD

Place the greens in a large bowl and top with the beans, chicken breast, and olive oil. Mix well before serving.

352 calories per serving. Each serving: P, SC, C, F.

MAIN DISHES

Simple Oven-Roasted Chicken Breast

Serves 2

This simple but delicious recipe is easy to double or quadruple to give you plenty of chicken you can use in sandwiches or other meals throughout the week. Feel free to swap in turkey breast if you prefer.

INGREDIENTS

2 boneless, skinless chicken breasts, about 3 ounces each

2 teaspoons olive oil

Pinch of sea salt

Pinch of black pepper

METHOD

1. Preheat the oven to 400°F with the rack in the middle position. Use a brush to brush a layer of olive oil onto a baking dish and one side of a sheet of parchment paper to prevent the chicken from sticking.
2. Brush the olive oil on the chicken breasts, and sprinkle with salt and pepper to taste.
3. Place the chicken breasts in the baking dish. Lay the parchment paper, oiled-side down, over the chicken. Tuck the edges into the pan and press the parchment down so that it's snug around the chicken. The chicken breasts should be completely covered with the parchment.
4. Transfer the chicken to the oven and bake until it's completely opaque all the way through and registers 165°F on an instant-read thermometer. Start checking after 15 minutes; total cooking time is usually 25 to 30 minutes. Serve the chicken immediately, or let it cool and refrigerate for up to a week.

150 calories per serving. Each serving: P, F.

Simple Pan-Roasted Turkey Breast

Serves 2

Pan-roasting is a simple, quick way to cook your proteins. Cooking times will vary, but you can use this method to cook poultry, meat, fish, or shellfish.

INGREDIENTS

2 boneless, skinless turkey breasts, about 3 ounces each

2 teaspoons olive oil

Pinch of sea salt

Pinch of black pepper

METHOD

1. Rub the turkey breasts with a small amount of olive oil and season with salt and pepper.
2. Heat the remaining oil in a medium-size skillet over medium heat. Place the turkey breasts in the skillet and cook, turning once, until cooked through, about 10 minutes.

127 calories per serving. Store in an airtight container in the refrigerator for up to 1 week. Each serving: P, F.

Carne Asada Tacos

Serves 2

Tacos don't have to ruin your healthy diet. These tacos satisfy your urge for Mexican food without all the extra fat and calories.

INGREDIENTS

2 teaspoons olive oil

½ cup diced yellow onion

2 cloves garlic, minced

1 jalapeño pepper, minced

2 teaspoons cumin

2 teaspoons coriander

Grated zest and juice of 2 limes

8 ounces skirt steak, sliced thinly

Pinch of sea salt

8 small corn tortillas

½ cup shredded cabbage

2 radishes, sliced

½ cup cilantro leaves, chopped

METHOD

1. Heat the oil in a large skillet over medium heat. Add the onion, garlic, jalapeño, cumin, and coriander; cook, stirring, until the onion is softened, about 30 seconds. Add the lime zest, juice, and skirt steak, and stir until the meat is cooked through, about 3 to 5 minutes. Remove from the heat and season with salt.

2. Warm the tortillas briefly to soften, either in the microwave for 10 seconds, or by waving carefully over a stovetop burner for 10 to 20 seconds. Place the tortillas on a serving plate and top each with an equal amount of meat, cabbage, radish, and cilantro. Serve immediately.

363 calories per serving. Each serving: P, SC, F.

Grilled Beefsteak with Caramelized Onions and Gorgonzola

Serves 2

Craving a steak? Choose a high-quality cut of meat and enjoy this delicious main course.

INGREDIENTS

8 ounces beef tenderloin steak (such as filet mignon)

Pinch of sea salt

Pinch of black pepper

2 tablespoons olive oil

1 medium yellow onion, sliced

½ cup water

2 tablespoons crumbled Gorgonzola cheese

METHOD

1. Preheat the grill or broiler to high. Season the beef with salt and pepper.

2. Heat the oil in a large sauté pan over medium heat. Add the onion and cook slowly, until softened. Add the water and another pinch of salt, and continue to cook until the water is reduced and the onion is golden and tender, about 20 minutes.

3. Place the beef on the grill and cook until caramelized, about 5 minutes on each side, or to your desired degree of doneness.

4. Transfer the steak to a serving plate, top with the onions and Gorgonzola, and serve immediately.

452 calories per serving. Each serving: P, 2 F.

Apple-Dijon Pork Chop

Serves 2

Meat has been paired with fruit since the Middle Ages—and for good reason. A sweet and tangy apple is the perfect counterbalance to any rich meat, especially pork. The type of apple used is completely up to you. Choose your favorite.

INGREDIENTS

2 4-ounce pork chops

Pinch of sea salt

Pinch of black pepper

2 teaspoons olive oil

½ cup chopped yellow onion

2 apples, peeled and sliced

2 cloves garlic, minced

2 tablespoons Dijon mustard

½ cup half-and-half

METHOD

1. Preheat the broiler or oven to high. Season the pork with salt and pepper, place in a small baking dish, and cook until golden and cooked through, about 5 minutes per side.

2. Meanwhile, heat the oil in a sauté pan over medium heat. Add the onion, apples, and garlic; cook, stirring, until the onion is tender and golden, about 3 to 5 minutes. Add the Dijon mustard and mix thoroughly, then stir in the half-and-half. Bring to a boil and cook for another minute, reducing the liquid to a thick sauce.

3. Place each broiled pork chop on a serving plate and cover with pan sauce. Season again with salt and pepper if you prefer, and serve immediately.

470 calories per serving. Each serving: P, C, F.

Buffalo Wings

Serves 2

This classic bar snack doesn't have to make you feel guilty. Here is a quick and easy version with just as much flavor, but half the calories.

INGREDIENTS

8 ounces chicken tenders

Pinch of sea salt

Pinch of black pepper

2 teaspoons unsalted butter

2 teaspoons white wine vinegar

2 teaspoons Worcestershire sauce

Pinch of cayenne pepper

Pinch of garlic powder

2 tablespoons Tabasco or other hot sauce

2 stalks celery, sliced in sticks

2 tablespoons nonfat Greek yogurt, for dipping

METHOD

1. Preheat the broiler or oven to high. Coat a small baking dish with parchment paper. Season the chicken tenders with salt and pepper, place them in the baking dish, and cook until golden on each side and cooked through, about 5 minutes per side.

2. Meanwhile, melt the butter in a small saucepan over medium heat. Stir in the vinegar, Worcestershire sauce, cayenne, garlic powder, and Tabasco. Bring to a boil and reduce for 1 minute to thicken.

3. When the chicken is cooked through, add it to the saucepan and toss to coat thoroughly. Transfer to a serving plate and garnish with the celery and yogurt. Serve immediately.

250 calories per serving. Each serving: P, F.

Grilled Greek Yogurt Chicken

Serves 2

Yogurt adds an appealing tang to this recipe, but, more important, the acid helps to tenderize and moisten a typically dry piece of meat. If you don't have a grill available, this recipe can be made easily in the oven or under the broiler.

INGREDIENTS

2 teaspoons olive oil

1 cup nonfat Greek yogurt

2 cloves garlic, minced

2 tablespoons chopped fresh oregano
    (or 2 teaspoons dried)

Grated zest of 2 lemons

2 4-ounce boneless and skinless chicken breasts

(*continued*)

METHOD

1. Preheat the grill to high. In a small bowl, stir together the oil, yogurt, garlic, oregano, and lemon zest. Coat the chicken breasts in this mixture, and place them on the preheated grill. Cook on high to mark each side with grill marks, about 3 to 5 minutes per side.

2. Then turn the heat to low, close the lid of the grill, and continue cooking until the meat is cooked through, about 5 to 8 more minutes. (The internal temperature of the chicken should be 165°F.) Serve with a third of a serving of Classic Greek Salad (see recipe, page 96) for a delicious, balanced meal.

268 calories per serving. Store leftovers in an airtight container in the refrigerator for up to 1 week. Each serving: P, C, F.

No-Guilt Pizza

Serves 2

You might initially turn your nose up at the idea of a cauliflower crust. But your mouth will set you straight as soon as you take a bite! This version has all the greatest elements of a pizza, without all the calories and fat. Prefer a veggie version? Swap in an assortment of vegetables along with the mushrooms instead of pepperoni.

INGREDIENTS

4 cloves garlic, sliced

2 tablespoons olive oil

4 cups grated or minced raw cauliflower

2 egg whites

2 teaspoons Italian seasoning

½ teaspoon sea salt

1 cup tomato sauce

½ cup nonfat mozzarella

6 mushrooms, sliced

20–24 pieces pepperoni

2 cups basil leaves, minced

METHOD

1. Preheat the oven to 400°F. Coat a baking sheet (or pizza pan) with pan spray. Combine the garlic and olive oil in a small bowl and set it aside.

2. Put the cauliflower in a microwave-safe bowl, cover tightly with plastic wrap, and heat for 3 to 5 minutes. Uncover and set aside to cool for 5 minutes.

3. Add the egg whites, Italian seasoning, and salt to the bowl with the cauliflower, and mix thoroughly. Turn the mixture out onto the prepared pan and pat it out into a circle about ½ inch thick. Bake for 20 to 30 minutes, until firm and golden on the edges.

4. Remove the cauliflower crust from the oven and spread it evenly with tomato sauce. Sprinkle nonfat mozzarella on top of the sauce, then evenly distribute the mushrooms, pepperoni, and basil leaves on top. Top with the reserved olive oil and garlic, then bake another 10 to 15 minutes, until golden and bubbly. Slice and scoop up with a pie-shaped spatula. Serve hot.

396 calories per serving. Each serving: P, 2 C, 2 F.

Steak Barcelona

Serves 2

Serve this dish with a starchy carb and steamed vegetables for a complete meal.

INGREDIENTS

6-ounce sirloin steak

Sea salt and black pepper to taste

1 medium yellow onion, sliced

2 cloves garlic, minced

1 tablespoon olive oil

1 cup low-sodium tomato sauce

1 tablespoon smoked paprika

1 large lemon, sliced

METHOD

1. Season the steak with salt and pepper to taste. In a sauté pan, sear the meat on both sides over high heat. Remove the steak to a plate and cover with foil.

2. In the same pan, sauté the onion and garlic in the olive oil over medium heat for 2 to 3 minutes until translucent. Add the tomato sauce and smoked paprika and turn the heat to low. Simmer uncovered for 5 to 7 minutes until slightly thickened.

3. Return the steak to the pan with the sauce, top with the sliced lemon, and simmer 5 minutes for medium-rare (longer for more well done).

231 calories per serving. Can store in an airtight container in the refrigerator for up to 1 week. Each serving: P, C, F.

Jerk Shrimp with Lime-Infused Pineapple

Serves 2

The sweetness of the pineapple balances the spices of this seafood dish.

INGREDIENTS

1 tablespoon paprika

½ teaspoon garlic powder

½ teaspoon cayenne pepper

¼ teaspoon ground thyme

⅛ teaspoon allspice

½ teaspoon see salt (or to taste)

8 ounces raw shrimp, peeled and deveined,
    tail off

1 cup cubed fresh pineapple

2 teaspoons lime zest

Juice of 1 lime

1 tablespoon canola oil

1 red bell pepper, cubed

4 scallions, sliced

METHOD

1. In a small bowl, blend the dry spices. Toss the raw shrimp in the spice mix and set aside.
2. Blend the cubed pineapple with the lime zest and juice.
3. In a large sauté pan or wok, sauté the shrimp in the canola oil for 2 to 3 minutes, just until it turns pink. Remove from the pan and add the bell pepper and scallions. Sauté for 2 to 3 minutes and return the shrimp to the pan. Add the marinated pineapple and heat through. Serve immediately.

218 calories per serving. Each serving: P, C, F.

Crispy Baked Fish and Kale

Serves 2

The crust on the fish gives this dish a unique twist.

INGREDIENTS

3 cups kale, washed, stems removed

1 tablespoon olive oil

1 tablespoon minced garlic

1 teaspoon lemon pepper

½ cup nonfat Greek yogurt

2 tablespoons Dijon mustard, coarse if preferred

1 teaspoon sea salt

½ teaspoon black pepper

2 4-ounce whitefish fillets (cod, pollack, etc.)

½ cup panko bread crumbs

METHOD

1. Preheat the oven to 400°F. In a large plastic bag, toss the kale with the olive oil, garlic, and lemon pepper. Spread the seasoned kale on a large baking sheet, leaving space in the center for the fish.

2. In a medium bowl, mix the yogurt, mustard, and salt and pepper. Place the fish fillets in the center of the baking sheet and spread the yogurt mixture on top. Gently press the panko bread crumbs on top of the yogurt mixture, forming a crust.

3. Roast for 10 to 12 minutes until the kale is crispy and the fish flakes easily. Serve immediately.

180 calories per serving. Each serving: P, C, F.

Baked Salmon and Asparagus Bundles

Serves 2

This simple yet delicious recipe is a great way to get more fish into your diet. Feel free to use other types of fish as you prefer.

INGREDIENTS

1 medium red onion, sliced thin

½ pound fresh asparagus spears, thinner stalks preferred

2 4-ounce raw salmon fillets, skin removed

Sea salt and black pepper to taste

2 cloves garlic, minced

Lemon slices

½ cup whole grape tomatoes

2 tablespoons fresh dill (or 1 teaspoon dried dill)

1 tablespoon olive oil

(*continued*)

METHOD

1. Preheat the oven to 400°F. Take two pieces of aluminum foil and place half of the sliced red onion and asparagus spears on each.

2. Season the salmon with the salt and pepper and place one fillet on top of each vegetable portion. Top with the garlic and lemon slices. Add the grape tomatoes and dill. Drizzle with olive oil.

3. Bring the sides of the foil together over the top and seal tightly with seams on top. Place the bundles on a baking sheet and roast for 10 to 12 minutes, until the fish flakes easily. Serve immediately.

310 calories per serving. Each serving: P, C, F.

Buffalo Turkey Lettuce Wraps

Serves 2

Love the flavor of Buffalo spices? Try this tasty twist.

INGREDIENTS

8 ounces raw turkey breast, cut in strips

1 tablespoon olive or canola oil

1 medium onion, sliced thin

1 red bell pepper, sliced thin

½ cup water chestnuts, sliced

½ cup Buffalo sauce (Frank's preferred)

1 teaspoon sriracha sauce (optional)

½ teaspoon garlic powder

½ teaspoon celery salt

6 large romaine or Bibb lettuce leaves, washed

1 teaspoon chopped peanuts

METHOD

1. In a large skillet, sauté the turkey breast in the oil until it's no longer pink, about 5 to 10 minutes.

2. Add the onion, pepper, and water chestnuts and cook for 3 to 5 minutes until tender. Add the Buffalo sauce, sriracha, garlic powder, and celery salt. Simmer, uncovered, 8 to 10 minutes.

3. Serve on lettuce leaves, wrapping up like tortillas. Garnish with peanuts. Serve immediately.

253 calories per serving. Each serving: P, C, F.

Beef Noodle Pho

Serves 2

This savory, broth-based soup can easily be prepared as a vegetarian version if you prefer. Replace the beef broth with a vegetable broth, and add 4 ounces of diced firm tofu in place of the beef.

INGREDIENTS

2 teaspoons coconut oil

1 cup diced yellow onion

½ cup diced carrot

2 tablespoons freshly grated gingerroot

½ teaspoon five-spice powder

2 teaspoons soy sauce

2 teaspoons Thai fish sauce

2 cups low-sodium beef broth

4 ounces dried rice noodles

4 ounces sirloin steak or London broil (placed in freezer for 30 minutes to make slicing easier)

2 tablespoons chopped scallion

1 cup bean sprouts

½ cup cilantro leaves

2 teaspoons sriracha

2 wedges of lime

METHOD

1. Heat the coconut oil in a large soup pot over medium-high heat. Add the onion, carrot, and ginger, and cook, stirring, until tender and slightly browned. Add the spice, soy sauce, fish sauce, and broth. Bring to a simmer, and cook on low heat for 10 to 30 minutes to infuse the flavors.

2. Bring a second pot of water to a boil. Add the rice noodles, cook for 2 to 3 minutes, then remove and set aside in cold water to prevent the noodles from cooking further.

3. Slice beef into thin strips. In a serving bowl, combine the sliced beef, scallion, bean sprouts, cilantro, and noodles. Bring the broth to a full boil, then immediately strain it into the soup bowl. This will cook the thinly sliced beef. Serve immediately topped with sriracha and lime.

411 calories per serving. Each serving: P, SC, C, F.

Part Three

Train to Get Cut

In the first three chapters, you learned about the importance of building and retaining lean muscle. Now let's get into *how* you do it.

The following section of the book shares the exercise component of The Cut. Chapter 7 includes the actual Cut workouts for beginner, intermediate, and advanced exercisers to help you shed body fat and build metabolically active muscle. You'll exercise between three and five times a week, depending on your fitness level. (See the beginning of chapter 7 for how to determine how often you'll work out.)

The following chapters describe the actual exercises that make up the workouts. You'll find boot camp cardio exercises in chapter 8 and weight-training exercises for different body parts in chapters 9 through 14.

To use this section, first look up the workouts you'll be doing in chapter 7. Then look up the exercise moves for each workout and make sure you know how to perform them properly. It's smart to keep an exercise log or journal to track your workouts. You can write down how many reps you were able to do, how much weight you lifted (if you're using dumbbells or gym exercise machines), and how you felt during and after your workouts. Seeing how many workouts you've already put in, and how you're progressing, can be a big motivator on days you're tempted to skip your workout.

7 The Cut Workouts

In the following chapters, you'll learn about different exercises that target different body parts. Now it's time to pull it all together! During the 12-week Cut program, you'll follow the diet as closely as you can. You'll also follow the exercise plans we've designed to help fit every reader's individual fitness goals.

In this chapter, you'll find the exercise plans for beginner, intermediate, and advanced exercisers. How do you know which plan is right for you?

- You'll do the **beginner** plan if you're new to working out, or haven't been exercising regularly for the last six months or so, and have little strength-training experience.
- You'll do the **intermediate** plan if you already exercise at least two or three times a week and have some strength-training experience.
- You'll do the **advanced** plan if you already exercise at least four times a week and have some experience with strength training.

You'll find two types of workouts in this chapter: body-weight, or home, exercise plans, and gym plans. The body-weight plans, as their names imply, include many body-weight exercises and other moves that require minimal equipment. (You will need a few sets of dumbbells.) The boot camp cardio part of the body-weight plan includes exercises that can be done at home—indoors or outside—with no equipment.

Prefer to work out at the gym? You'll find exercises that use popular gym equipment, and you can do your cardio sessions on the treadmill, elliptical, stair machine, or stationary bicycle. Another advantage to using these pieces of equipment is that you can use the timer to keep track of your intervals. As you get fitter, you should see your interval speed increase.

For Beginners Only

We designed these plans to provide options for just about anyone who works out. It's important to note, though, that if you opt for the beginner plan, you won't exercise as often, or as intensely, as on the other two plans. That means that you'll expend fewer calories through exercise, so it's important to stick to the Cut meal plan to lose a significant amount of weight.

If you fit into the beginner category but want to be sure you're burning enough calories to lose a dramatic amount of weight, you can do additional cardio exercise—like walking or biking—if you like. You needn't push yourself during these workouts; your goal is to just burn a few more calories for enhanced fat loss.

A few more things to keep in mind before you start your exercise plan. First off, make sure you warm up before you start lifting weights. Walk in place or walk on a treadmill for 3 to 5 minutes to elevate your heart rate and increase blood flow throughout your body. Use that time to mentally gear up for your workout.

When doing an exercise that requires weights or a weight machine at the gym, choose a weight that is light enough that you can do the exercise for as long as you're supposed to (or for the assigned number of reps), but heavy enough that the last few reps are challenging. In other words, if you can bench-press a weight 20 times, it's too light. If you can only do, say, 8 reps, it's too heavy. The key is to choose a weight with which you can complete the assigned number of reps, in good form—and that you feel challenged while doing so.

That being said, if you're new to lifting weights, don't worry if you can't complete all of the reps of an exercise when you start out. You'll quickly get stronger and more comfortable with the exercises, and by the third or fourth week, you should already notice a difference in your ability to complete the exercises. Feel free to use a heavier weight whenever you're ready. The key is to continually keep challenging yourself.

From Obi:

You can't out-train a bad diet. Proper nutrition is just as important for overall weight loss!

The Importance of Rest

You know that exercise burns calories. You're motivated to lose weight, and that means burning more calories than you take in. So you may be thinking, *Why not exercise more often? Why not work out six or even seven days a week?*

First off, over-exercising is counterproductive. It's better to exercise intensely three to five days a week (depending on your current fitness level and goals) than to exercise nearly every day of the week. When you strength-train, you create micro-tears in your body's muscles that are repaired over the next 48 hours. That process of repairing is actually when you get stronger! Exercise too often and you interfere with that process.

Exercising too often also increases your risk of getting injured. You're more likely to be fatigued, which means you can't work out as intensely when you're supposed to. So do your body a favor—follow the exercise plan, and have confidence that it will work for you! That's what it's been designed to do.

Okay, you know which exercise plan to choose. You know to warm up before you start lifting weights. You know how much weight to lift. So let's get after it!

The 10-Minute Workout

Don't have time to do a full workout, but still want to get your heart rate up, get leaner, and lose body fat? Give one of these quick workouts a try:

- 2 sets of push-ups (10 to 12 reps); followed by 2 sets of dips (10 to 12 reps); followed by 2 sets of high knees (15 seconds each set); and 2 sets of mountain climbers (15 seconds each set).
- Choose one exercise from each body part chapter for a total body workout. You might do squats from the leg chapter; bent-over rows from the back chapter; push-ups from the chest chapter; shoulder presses from the shoulder chapter; biceps curls and triceps kickbacks from the arm chapter; and crunches from the ab chapter. You'll work all of your major muscle groups in less than 10 minutes!

BEGINNER HOME EXERCISE PLAN

Week 1 to Week 6

You'll exercise 3 times a week, lifting weights and then doing the boot camp cardio exercises. (If the Monday/Wednesday/Friday routine doesn't work for you, feel free to do Sunday/Tuesday/Thursday or another schedule. Just give yourself two days between sessions.)

Warm up for 3 to 5 minutes before you start lifting weights. You will rest briefly between each strength exercise (for 15 to 25 seconds). You will walk slowly as active rest between the boot camp cardio exercises.

Circuit-Training Program

On Monday, Wednesday, and Friday, **do 3 sets** of this circuit, followed by the boot camp cardio routine. Perform each strength exercise in order, rest for 15 to 25 seconds, move on to the next strength exercise, and so on:

Shoulder presses (page 184): 12 to 15 reps
   15 to 25 seconds rest
Push-ups or modified push-ups (page 165): 12 to 15 reps
   15 to 25 seconds rest
Body-weight squats (page 155): 12 to 15 reps
   15 to 25 seconds rest
Triceps kickbacks (page 178): 12 to 15 reps
   15 to 25 seconds rest
Planks (page 193): hold for 30 seconds (or as long as you can)
   15 to 25 seconds rest
Bent-over rows (page 171): 12 to 15 reps
   15 to 25 seconds rest

Boot Camp Cardio Routine

After the circuits, **do 3 cycles** of the following boot camp cardio routine:

High knees (page 149): 15 seconds
　Run or walk in place for 15 to 30 seconds
Jumping jacks (page 146): 15 seconds
　Run or walk in place for 15 to 30 seconds
Basketball jump shots (page 153): 15 seconds
　Run or walk in place for 15 to 30 seconds
Mountain climbers (page 146): 15 seconds
　Run or walk in place for 15 to 30 seconds
Run around the towel (page 151): 15 seconds
　Run or walk in place for 15 to 30 seconds
Squat uppercuts (page 150): 15 seconds
　Run or walk in place for 15 to 30 seconds

From Obi:

The mental element of staying in shape is just as important as how you eat and exercise. Embrace a fit, healthy mind-set and your behavior will follow.

Week 7 to Week 12

Circuit-Training Program

You'll continue to exercise 3 times a week, lifting weights and then doing the boot camp cardio exercises. You will rest briefly between each strength exercise (for 15 to 25 seconds). You will walk slowly as active rest between the boot camp cardio exercises.

On Monday, Wednesday, and Friday, **do 3 sets** of this circuit before doing the boot camp cardio routine:

Biceps curls (page 179): 12 to 15 reps
    15 to 25 seconds rest
Wall sits (page 156): 12 to 15 reps
    15 to 25 seconds rest
Push-ups (page 165): 12 to 15 reps
    15 to 25 seconds rest
Body-weight calf raises (page 158): 12 to 15 reps
    15 to 25 seconds rest
In and outs (page 196): 12 to 15 reps
    15 to 25 seconds rest
Dips (page 177): 12 to 15 reps
    15 to 25 seconds rest

Boot Camp Cardio Routine

After the circuits, **do 4 cycles** of the boot camp cardio routine:

Basketball jump shots (page 153): 15 seconds
    Run or walk in place for 15 to 30 seconds
Jumping jacks (page 146): 15 seconds
    Run or walk in place for 15 to 30 seconds
Suicides (page 152): 15 seconds
    Run or walk in place for 15 to 30 seconds
Burpees (page 147): 15 seconds
    Run or walk in place for 15 to 30 seconds
Switch feet (page 152): 15 seconds
    Run or walk in place for 15 to 30 seconds
Quick feet (page 150): 15 seconds
    Run or walk in place for 15 to 30 seconds

BEGINNER GYM EXERCISE PLAN

Week 1 to Week 6

You'll exercise 3 times a week, lifting weights and then doing cardio. (If the Monday/Wednesday/Friday routine doesn't work for you, feel free to do Sunday/Tuesday/Thursday or another schedule. Just give yourself two days between sessions.)

Warm up for 3 to 5 minutes before you start lifting weights. When you do a superset, do all of the exercises of the superset before resting for 15 to 25 seconds, then starting the next exercise.

Circuit-Training Program

On Monday, Wednesday, and Friday, **do 3 sets** of the circuit for the day, followed by cardio:

Monday

Biceps/back superset (1 biceps exercise followed by 1 back exercise; repeat)
Biceps exercises
    Preacher curls (page 181): 12 to 15 reps
    Seated hammer curls (page 182): 12 to 15 reps
Back exercises
    Seated low rows (page 174): 12 to 15 reps
    Lat pull-downs (page 173): 12 to 15 reps
Cardio
    You can use any piece of cardio equipment for this part of the workout—elliptical, stair machine, treadmill, or exercise bike.
    If you use the treadmill, warm up for 5 minutes at 3.0 mph, or a pace that feels easy to you. For the next 15 minutes, do the following intervals:
    Walk at 3.0 mph for 30 seconds; then jog at 6.0 mph for 30 seconds; repeat for 15 minutes. (If 6.0 mph is too fast for you, choose a speed that makes you feel uncomfortable; the key is to be out of breath and pushing yourself during the faster part of the interval.)

If you use a different piece of equipment, warm up at an easy pace for 5 minutes, and follow the same 30 seconds/30 seconds intervals. The recovery interval should be at an easy pace; the challenging interval should be at a pace that feels uncomfortable. Do the intervals for 15 minutes, for a total of 20 minutes including the warm-up.

From Morris:

I don't like to do cardio, but I accept I have to do it. I'd much rather play basketball than get on a machine. If I can't play ball, though, I'll get on either the treadmill, elliptical, or stair machine. I mix it up so I'm not doing the same machine every day.

Making the Cut: Real People, Real Results

Name: Joey Ray
Age: 45
Location: Lodi, California
Occupation: Teacher
Height: 5'6"
Starting weight: 215 pounds
Ending weight: 198 pounds

On The Cut, I felt the weight come off right away. I noticed a difference in my body in the first couple of weeks, which motivated me to keep working hard.

I'm a single mother, so I got up at 5:00 a.m. to do the weight portion of the workout and then did cardio after work. I loved the cardio intervals because they went by fast! I enjoyed seeing my progress and being able to go faster and faster on the treadmill, too.

> I loved the cardio intervals because they went by fast! I enjoyed seeing my progress and being able to go faster and faster on the treadmill, too.

Today I feel really good and I feel strong—the program has me motivated to keep eating healthy and keep going to the gym. I would definitely recommend the program; it really works and the meals are easy to follow. And my students have noticed my weight loss, too. They tell me, "Miss Ray, all of your clothes are getting super-baggy!"

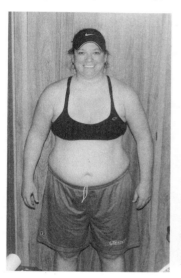 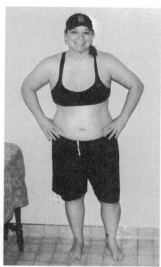

Wednesday

Chest/triceps/ab superset (1 chest move, 1 triceps move, 1 ab move; repeat)

Chest exercises

Push-ups or modified push-ups (page 165): 12 to 15 reps

Incline chest presses (page 168): 12 to 15 reps

Triceps exercises

Triceps push-downs (page 180): 12 to 15 reps

Dips (page 177): 12 to 15 reps

Ab exercises

Planks (page 193): hold for 25 seconds

Leg raises (using Roman chair) (page 199): 20 reps

Cardio

Do 20 minutes of cardio, following the same 5-minute warm-up and 15 minutes of 30 seconds/30 seconds intervals you did on Monday.

Friday

Leg/shoulder supersets (2 leg exercises, 1 shoulder exercise; repeat)

Leg exercises

Body-weight squats (page 155): 12 to 15 reps

Leg extensions (page 160): 12 to 15 reps

Prone leg curls (page 163): 12 to 15 reps

Calf raises on leg press machine (page 161): 12 to 15 reps

Shoulder exercises

Shoulder presses (page 184): 12 to 15 reps

Front raises (page 186): 12 to 15 reps

Cardio

Do 20 minutes of cardio, following the same 5-minute warm-up and 15 minutes of 30 seconds/30 seconds intervals you did on Monday.

Week 7 to Week 12

Circuit-Training Program

On Monday, Wednesday, and Friday, **do 3 sets** of the circuit for the day, followed by cardio:

Monday

Leg exercises

Leg presses (page 159): 10 to 12 reps

Wall sits (page 156): 25 seconds

Leg extensions (page 160): 10 to 12 reps

Calf raises on leg press machine (page 161): 10 to 12 reps

Cardio

Do 20 minutes of cardio, following the same 5-minute warm-up and 15 minutes of 30 seconds/30 seconds intervals as during week 1 to week 6.

Wednesday

Chest/biceps/triceps superset (1 chest exercise, 1 biceps exercise, 1 triceps exercise; repeat)

Chest presses (page 167): 10 to 12 reps

Cable biceps curls (page 181): 10 to 12 reps

Triceps push-downs (page 180): 10 to 12 reps

Rest no more than 30 seconds before **doing 3 sets** of these ab moves:

Ab exercises

Sit-ups (page 197): 15 to 20 reps

Bicycles (page 195): 20 reps

Cardio

Do 20 minutes of cardio, following the same 5-minute warm-up and 15 minutes of 30 seconds/30 seconds intervals as during week 1 to week 6.

Friday

Shoulder/back superset (1 shoulder exercise, 1 back exercise; repeat)

Shoulder exercises

Upright rows (page 185): 10 to 12 reps

Lateral raises (page 185): 10 to 12 reps

Back exercises

T-bar rows (page 174): 10 to 12 reps

Lat pull-downs (page 173): 10 to 12 reps

Cardio

Do 20 minutes of cardio, following the same 5-minute warm-up and 15 minutes of 30 seconds/30 seconds intervals as during week 1 to week 6.

INTERMEDIATE HOME EXERCISE PLAN

Week 1 to Week 6

You'll exercise 4 times a week, lifting weights and then doing the boot camp cardio exercises. (If the Monday/Tuesday/Thursday/Friday routine doesn't work for you, feel free to choose another schedule. Just give yourself two days off after the first two days of lifting.)

Warm up for 3 to 5 minutes before you start lifting weights. You will rest briefly between each strength exercise (for 15 to 25 seconds). You will run or walk as active rest between the boot camp cardio exercises.

Circuit-Training Program

On Monday, Tuesday, Thursday, and Friday, **do 3 sets** of the circuit, followed by the boot camp cardio routine. Perform each strength exercise in order, rest for 15 to 25 seconds, move on to the next strength exercise, and so on:

Wall sits (page 156): 45 seconds
   15 to 25 seconds rest
Front raises (page 186): 10 to 12 reps
   15 to 25 seconds rest
Triceps kickbacks (page 178): 10 to 12 reps
   15 to 25 seconds rest
Bent-over rows (page 171): 10 to 12 reps
   15 to 25 seconds rest
Push-ups (page 165): 10 to 12 reps
   15 to 25 seconds rest
Seated hammer curls (page 182): 10 to 12 reps
   15 to 25 seconds rest
Dips (page 177): 10 to 12 reps
   15 to 25 seconds rest

Boot Camp Cardio Routine

On Monday, Tuesday, Thursday, and Friday, after the circuits, **do 4 cycles** of this boot camp cardio routine:

Burpees (page 147): 20 seconds

    Run or walk in place for 15 to 25 seconds

Suicides (page 152): 20 seconds

    Run or walk in place for 15 to 25 seconds

Jumping jacks (page 146): 20 seconds

    Run or walk in place for 15 to 25 seconds

Basketball jump shots (page 153): 20 seconds

    Run or walk in place for 15 to 25 seconds

Squat uppercuts (page 150): 20 seconds

    Run or walk in place for 15 to 25 seconds

Ski jumps (page 148): 20 seconds

    Run or walk in place for 15 to 25 seconds

High knees (page 149): 20 seconds

    Run or walk in place for 15 to 25 seconds

Week 7 to Week 12

Circuit-Training Program

On Monday, Tuesday, Thursday, and Friday, **do 3 sets** of the circuit, followed by the boot camp cardio routine:

Incline push-ups (on bench or box) (page 166): 10 to 12 reps

    15 to 25 seconds rest

Body-weight squats (page 155): 10 to 12 reps

    15 to 25 seconds rest

Triceps kickbacks (page 178): 10 to 12 reps

    15 to 25 seconds rest

Seated hammer curls (page 182): 10 to 12 reps

    15 to 25 seconds rest

Bent-over rows (page 171): 10 to 12 reps

    15 to 25 seconds rest

Body-weight calf raises (page 158): 10 to 12 reps
   15 to 25 seconds rest
Lunges (page 157): 10 to 12 reps
   15 to 25 seconds rest

Boot Camp Cardio Routine

On Monday, Tuesday, Thursday, and Friday, after the circuits, **do 4 cycles** of the boot camp cardio routine:

High knees (page 149): 20 seconds
   Run or walk in place for 15 to 25 seconds
Mountain climbers (page 146): 20 seconds
   Run or walk in place for 15 to 25 seconds
Basketball jump shots (page 153): 20 seconds
   Run or walk in place for 15 to 25 seconds
Burpees (page 147): 20 seconds
   Run or walk in place for 15 to 25 seconds
Jumping jacks (page 146): 20 seconds
   Run or walk in place for 15 to 25 seconds
Ski jumps (page 148): 20 seconds
   Run or walk in place for 15 to 25 seconds
Quick feet (page 150): 20 seconds
   Run or walk in place for 15 to 25 seconds

INTERMEDIATE GYM EXERCISE PLAN

Week 1 to Week 6

You'll exercise 4 times a week, lifting weights and then doing cardio. (If the Monday/ Tuesday/Thursday/Friday routine doesn't work for you, feel free to choose another schedule. Just maintain the same timing and days off.)

Warm up for 3 to 5 minutes before you start lifting weights. When you do a superset, do all of the exercises of the superset before resting for 15 to 25 seconds, then starting the next exercise.

Circuit-Training Program

On Monday, Tuesday, Thursday, and Friday, **do 3 sets** of the circuit for the day, followed by cardio:

Monday

Chest/triceps superset (1 chest exercise, 1 triceps exercise; repeat)
Chest exercises
   Chest presses (page 167): 10 to 12 reps
   Upright flies (page 169): 10 to 12 reps
   Incline push-ups on bench (page 166): 10 to 12 reps
Triceps exercises
   Triceps kickbacks (page 178): 10 to 12 reps
   Triceps push-downs (page 180): 10 to 12 reps
   Triceps push-ups (page 178): 10 to 12 reps

Tuesday

Leg/ab superset (2 leg exercises, 1 ab exercise; repeat)
Leg exercises
   Smith machine squats (page 162): 10 to 12 reps
   Leg extensions (page 160): 10 to 12 reps
   Body-weight calf raises (page 158): 15 to 20 reps
   Prone leg curls (page 163): 10 to 12 reps
   Lunges (page 157): 10 to 12 reps
   Calf raises on leg press machine (page 161): 15 to 20 reps
Ab exercises
   Leg raises (using Roman chair) (page 199): 20 reps
   Crunches (page 196): 20 reps
   Kneeling cable crunches (page 198): 20 reps

Thursday

Shoulder exercises

Seated shoulder presses (page 189): 10 to 12 reps

Upright rows (page 185): 10 to 12 reps

Shoulder shrugs (page 187): 10 to 12 reps

Friday

Back/biceps superset (1 back exercise, 1 biceps exercise; repeat)

Back exercises

Pull-ups or lat pull-downs (pages 172 and 173): 10 to 12 reps

Seated low rows (page 174): 10 to 12 reps

Biceps exercises

Preacher curls (page 181): 10 to 12 reps

Cable biceps curls (page 181): 10 to 12 reps

Making the Cut: Real People, Real Results

Name: Tyrone Foster

Age: 45

Location: Simpsonville, South Carolina

Occupation: Truck driver

Height: 5'9"

Starting weight: 191 pounds

Ending weight: 170 pounds

I was super excited about starting The Cut; the only real challenge for me about the program was the cardio. I noticed a change in my weight within the first 5 days, and a change in my body at about the 30-day mark. But the biggest game changer is now I feel confident taking my shirt off at any time!

I really love the supersetting weight-lifting component of the program—it was kind of like getting a cardio session in with few to no rest periods.

To make following the diet easier, I would meal-prep three to four meals a week for me, and for my wife to take with her lunch. I always cooked extras for the family to eat dinner during the first part of the week. My family has been excited for me to do the program since day one; they've noticed a significant change in me as a whole man, not just the physical change. Over the holidays, my distant family noticed the difference in me, too—some of them didn't even recognize me!

I believe that this program has laid a solid foundation for my fitness journey. The changes I've made in my life not just physically but also emotionally, spiritually, and financially have been a great benefit to lifting my family to a higher level.

I can truly say that I have never, ever felt so good about my body…after the 12 weeks on The Cut, I feel really great about my progress and am looking forward to improving my physique even more through nutrition and exercise. I would recommend this program to anyone no matter what their fitness goals are!

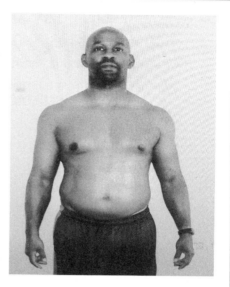

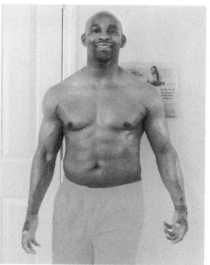

I really love the supersetting weight-lifting component of the program—it was kind of like getting a cardio session in with few to no rest periods.

Cardio (40 minutes)

You can use any piece of cardio equipment for this part of the workout—elliptical, stair machine, treadmill, or exercise bike.

If you use the treadmill, warm up for 7 minutes at 3.0 mph, or a pace that feels easy to you. For the next 33 minutes, do the following intervals:

Walk at 3.0 mph for 30 seconds; then jog at 7.0 mph for 30 seconds; repeat for 33 minutes. (If 7.0 mph is too fast for you, choose a speed that makes you feel somewhat uncomfortable; the key is to be out of breath and pushing yourself during the faster part of the interval.)

If you use a different piece of equipment, warm up at an easy pace for 7 minutes, and follow the same 30 seconds/30 seconds intervals for 33 minutes, for a total of 40 minutes including the warm-up.

Week 7 to Week 12

Circuit-Training Program

On Monday, Tuesday, Thursday, and Friday, **do 3 sets** of the circuit for the day, followed by cardio:

Monday

Biceps/triceps superset (1 biceps exercise, 1 triceps exercise; repeat)

Biceps exercises

Seated hammer curls (page 182): 10 to 12 reps

Biceps curls (page 179): 10 to 12 reps

Triceps exercises

Triceps kickbacks (page 178): 10 to 12 reps

Triceps push-ups (page 178): 10 to 12 reps

After the supersets, **do 3 sets** of the following ab exercises:

Ab exercises

Sit-ups (page 197): 20 reps

Leg raises (using Roman chair) (page 199): 20 reps

Planks (page 193): 35 seconds each

Tuesday

Shoulder/back superset (1 shoulder exercise, 1 back exercise; repeat)

Shoulder exercises

Front raises (page 186): 10 to 12 reps

Upright rows (page 185): 10 to 12 reps

Lateral raises (page 185): 10 to 12 reps

Back exercises

Lat pull-downs (page 173): 10 to 12 reps

Seated low rows (page 174): 10 to 12 reps

T-bar rows (page 174): 10 to 12 reps

Thursday

Leg exercises

Smith machine squats (page 162): 10 to 12 reps

Leg presses (page 159): 10 to 12 reps

Prone leg curls (page 163): 10 to 12 reps

Leg extensions (page 160): 10 to 12 reps

Body-weight calf raises (page 158): 10 to 12 reps

Calf raises on leg press machine (page 161): 10 to 12 reps

Friday

Chest/ab superset (1 chest exercise, 1 ab exercise; repeat)

Chest exercises

Push-ups (page 165): 10 to 12 reps

Incline chest presses (page 168): 10 to 12 reps

Upright flies (using butterfly chest machine) (page 169): 10 to 12 reps

Ab exercises

In and outs (page 196): 25 reps

Bicycles (page 195): 25 reps

Sit-ups (page 197): 25 reps

Cardio (40 minutes)

Do the same cardio routine that you did during week 1 to week 6; warm up for 7 minutes at 3.0 mph, or a pace that feels easy to you. For the next 33 minutes, do 30 seconds/30 seconds intervals at 7.0 mph or another pace that feels somewhat uncomfortable, for a total of 40 minutes including warm-up.

ADVANCED HOME EXERCISE PLAN

Week 1 to Week 6

You'll exercise 5 times a week, lifting weights and then doing the boot camp cardio exercises. (If the Monday/Tuesday/Wednesday/Thursday/Friday routine doesn't work for you, feel free to choose another schedule. Just give yourself two days of rest each week, which may or may not be consecutive.)

Warm up for 3 to 5 minutes before you start lifting weights. You will rest briefly between each strength exercise (for 15 to 25 seconds). You will run or walk as active rest between the boot camp cardio exercises.

Circuit-Training Program

On Monday, Tuesday, Wednesday, Thursday, and Friday, **do 5 sets** of the circuit, followed by the boot camp cardio routine. Perform each strength exercise in order, rest for 15 to 25 seconds, move on to the next strength exercise, and so on:

Shoulder presses (page 184): 10 to 12 reps

Rest 15 to 25 seconds

Push-ups or modified push-ups (page 165): 10 to 12 reps

Rest 15 to 25 seconds

Biceps curls (page 179): 10 to 12 reps
    Rest 15 to 25 seconds
Wall sits (page 156): 60 seconds
    Rest 15 to 25 seconds
Triceps kickbacks (page 178): 10 to 12 reps
    Rest 15 to 25 seconds
Lunges (page 157): 10 to 12 reps
    Rest 15 to 25 seconds
Bent-over rows (page 171): 10 to 12 reps
    Rest 15 to 25 seconds
Body-weight squats (page 155): 10 to 12 reps
    Rest 15 to 25 seconds

Boot Camp Cardio Routine

On Monday, Tuesday, Wednesday, Thursday, and Friday, after the circuits, **do 6 cycles** of the boot camp cardio routine:

Suicides (page 152): 30 seconds
    Run or walk in place for 15 to 25 seconds
High knees (page 149): 30 seconds
    Run or walk in place for 15 to 25 seconds
Mountain climbers (page 146): 30 seconds
    Run or walk in place for 15 to 25 seconds
Jumping jacks (page 146): 30 seconds
    Run or walk in place for 15 to 25 seconds
Basketball jump shots (page 153): 30 seconds
    Run or walk in place for 15 to 25 seconds
Ski jumps (page 148): 30 seconds
    Run or walk in place for 15 to 25 seconds
Burpees (page 147): 30 seconds
    Run or walk in place for 15 to 25 seconds
Quick feet (page 150): 30 seconds
    Run or walk in place for 15 to 25 seconds

Week 7 to Week 12

Circuit-Training Program

On Monday, Tuesday, Wednesday, Thursday, and Friday, **do 5 sets** of the circuit, followed by the boot camp cardio routine:

Dips (page 177): 10 to 12 reps
  Rest 15 to 25 seconds
Lunges (page 157): 10 to 12 reps
  Rest 15 to 25 seconds
Bent-over rows (page 171): 10 to 12 reps
  Rest 15 to 25 seconds
Upright rows (page 185): 10 to 12 reps
  Rest 15 to 25 seconds
Biceps curls (page 179): 10 to 12 reps
  Rest 15 to 25 seconds
Body-weight squats (page 155): 10 to 12 reps
  Rest 15 to 25 seconds
Push-ups or modified push-ups (page 165): 10 to 12 reps
  Rest 15 to 25 seconds
Body-weight calf raises (page 158): 10 to 12 reps
  Rest 15 to 25 seconds

Boot Camp Cardio Routine

On Monday, Tuesday, Wednesday, Thursday, and Friday, after the circuits, **do 6 cycles** of these moves:

Jumping jacks (page 146): 30 seconds
  Run or walk in place for 15 to 25 seconds
Burpees (page 147): 30 seconds
  Run or walk in place for 15 to 25 seconds

Ski jumps (page 148): 30 seconds

Run or walk in place for 15 to 25 seconds

Basketball jump shots (page 153): 30 seconds

Run or walk in place for 15 to 25 seconds

High knees (page 149): 30 seconds

Run or walk in place for 15 to 25 seconds

Switch feet (page 152): 30 seconds

Run or walk in place for 15 to 25 seconds

Mountain climbers (page 146): 30 seconds

Run or walk in place for 15 to 25 seconds

Quick feet (page 150): 30 seconds

Run or walk in place for 15 to 25 seconds

Making the Cut: Real People, Real Results

Name: Stacy Ezel

Age: 46

Location: Phoenix, Arizona

Occupation: Real estate

Height: 6'0"

Starting weight: 206 pounds

Ending weight: 188 pounds

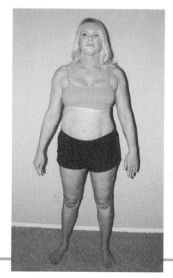

I wanted to try The Cut because I wanted to be able to look in the mirror and be proud of myself. My weight's been an issue for the last three years or so, and I have tried other diets before. The diets would work for a little bit, but then I would lose focus or get bored with the program. Plus the nutritional guidelines were too general.

I was excited and nervous at the same time to start The Cut, and I noticed a difference in my body in the first two weeks. With a more positive direction and overall nutrition plan, I now feel empowered to do better for myself, my body, my health, and my future.

I was excited and nervous at the same time to start The Cut, and I noticed a difference in my body in the first two weeks.

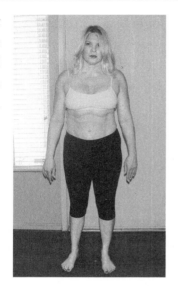

ADVANCED GYM EXERCISE PLAN

Week 1 to Week 6

You'll exercise 5 times a week, lifting weights and then doing cardio. (If the Monday/Tuesday/Wednesday/Thursday/Friday routine doesn't work for you, feel free to choose another schedule. Just maintain the same timing and take two days of rest during the week.)

Warm up for 3 to 5 minutes before you start lifting weights. When you do a superset, do all of the exercises of the superset before resting for 15 to 25 seconds, then starting the next exercise.

Circuit-Training Program

On Monday through Friday, **do 4 sets** of the circuit routine for the day, followed by cardio:

Monday

Chest/biceps superset (1 chest exercise, 1 biceps exercise; repeat)

Chest exercises

Chest presses (page 167): 10 to 12 reps

Upright flies (using butterfly chest machine) (page 169): 10 to 12 reps

Push-ups (page 165): 10 to 12 reps

Biceps exercises

Biceps curls (page 179): 10 to 12 reps

Preacher curls (page 181): 10 to 12 reps

Cable biceps curls (page 181): 10 to 12 reps

After the supersets, **do 4 sets** of the following ab exercises:

Ab exercises

Sit-ups (page 197): 30 reps

Leg raises (using Roman chair) (page 199): 30 reps

Kneeling cable crunches (page 198): 30 reps

Tuesday

Leg/triceps supersets (2 leg exercises, 1 triceps exercise; repeat)

Leg exercises

Smith machine squats (page 162): 10 to 12 reps

Lunges (page 157): 10 to 12 reps

Leg extensions (page 160): 10 to 12 reps

Body-weight calf raises (page 158): 15 to 20 reps

Prone leg curls (page 163): 10 to 12 reps

Calf raises on leg press machine (page 161): 30 reps

Triceps exercises

Dips (page 177): 10 to 12 reps

Triceps kickbacks (page 178): 10 to 12 reps

Triceps push-downs (page 180): 10 to 12 reps

Wednesday

Shoulder/back superset (1 shoulder exercise, 1 back exercise; repeat)

Shoulder exercises

Shoulder presses (page 184): 10 to 12 reps

Front raises (page 186): 10 to 12 reps

Upright rows (page 185): 10 to 12 reps

Shoulder shrugs (page 187): 10 to 12 reps

Back exercises

Pull-ups (page 172): 10 to 12 reps

Lat pull-downs (page 173): 10 to 12 reps

T-bar rows (page 174): 10 to 12 reps

Bent-over rows (page 171): 10 to 12 reps

After the supersets, **do 4 sets** of the following ab exercises:

Ab exercises

Crunches (page 196): 30 reps

Scissors (page 195): 30 reps

Planks (page 193): 60 seconds each

Thursday

Chest/biceps superset (1 chest exercise, 1 biceps exercise; repeat)

Chest exercises

Chest presses (page 167): 10 to 12 reps

Upright flies (using butterfly chest machine) (page 169): 10 to 12 reps

Incline push-ups (page 166): 15 to 20 reps

Biceps exercises

Preacher curls (page 181): 10 to 12 reps

Biceps curls (page 179): 10 to 12 reps

Seated hammer curls (page 182): 10 to 12 reps

Friday

Ab exercises

Bicycles (page 195): 30 reps

In and outs (page 196): 30 reps

Sit-ups (page 197): 30 reps

Cardio (60 minutes)

You can use any piece of cardio equipment for this part of the workout—elliptical, stair machine, treadmill, or exercise bike.

If you use the treadmill, warm up for 15 minutes at 4.0 mph, or a pace that feels fairly easy to you. For the next 45 minutes, do the following intervals:

Walk or jog at 4.0 mph, then run at 7.0 to 8.0 mph for 30 seconds; repeat for 45 minutes. (If that speed is too fast for you, choose a speed that makes you feel somewhat uncomfortable; the key is to be out of breath and pushing yourself during the faster part of the interval.)

If you use a different piece of equipment, warm up at an easy pace for 15 minutes, and follow the same 30 seconds/30 seconds intervals for 45 minutes, for a total of 60 minutes including the warm-up.

Week 7 to Week 12

Circuit-Training Program

On Monday through Friday, **do 4 sets** of the circuit routine for the day, followed by cardio:

Monday

Leg/ab superset (1 leg exercise, 1 ab exercise; repeat. After the superset, do the remaining 4 leg exercises)

Leg exercises

Smith machine squats (page 162): 10 to 12 reps

Leg presses (page 159): 10 to 12 reps

Calf raises on leg press machine (page 161): 20 to 25 reps

Wall sits (page 156): 60 seconds each

Leg extensions (page 160): 10 to 12 reps

Prone leg curls (page 163): 10 to 12 reps

Body-weight calf raises (page 158): 20 to 25 reps

Ab exercises

Planks (page 193): 60 seconds each

Kneeling cable crunches (page 198): 30 seconds each

Leg raises (using Roman chair (page 199): 30 reps each

Tuesday

Chest/triceps supersets (1 chest exercise, 1 triceps exercise; repeat)

Chest exercises

Chest presses (page 167): 10 to 12 reps

Push-ups or modified push-ups (page 165): 10 to 12 reps

Incline chest presses (page 168): 10 to 12 reps

Upright flies (using butterfly chest machine) (page 169): 10 to 12 reps

Triceps exercises

Triceps push-downs (page 180): 10 to 12 reps

Dips (page 177): 10 to 12 reps

Triceps kickbacks (page 178): 10 to 12 reps

Triceps push-ups (page 178): 10 to 12 reps

Wednesday

Biceps/back superset (1 biceps exercise, 1 back exercise; repeat)

Biceps exercises

Biceps curls (page 179): 10 to 12 reps

Preacher curls (page 181): 10 to 12 reps

Seated hammer curls (page 182): 10 to 12 reps

Cable biceps curls (page 181): 10 to 12 reps

Back exercises

Seated low rows (page 174): 10 to 12 reps

T-bar rows (page 174): 10 to 12 reps

Bent-over rows (page 171): 10 to 12 reps

Lat pull-downs (page 173): 10 to 12 reps

Thursday

Shoulder exercises

Shoulder shrugs (page 187): 10 to 12 reps

Shoulder presses (page 184): 10 to 12 reps

Lateral raises (page 185): 10 to 12 reps

Front raises (page 186): 10 to 12 reps

Friday

Leg/ab superset (2 leg exercises, 1 ab exercise; repeat)

Leg exercises

Smith machine squats (page 162): 10 to 12 reps

Leg extensions (page 160): 10 to 12 reps

Calf raises on leg press machine (page 161): 20 to 25 reps

Prone leg curls (page 163): 10 to 12 reps

Body-weight calf raises (page 158): 20 to 25 reps

Ab exercises

In and outs (page 196): 30 reps

Leg raises (using Roman chair) (page 199): 30 reps

Crunches (page 196): 30 reps

Cardio

Five days a week, after the weight-lifting routine, do the same cardio routine that you did week 1 through week 6: Warm up for 15 minutes at 4.0 mph, or a pace that feels fairly easy to you. For the next 45 minutes, do 30 seconds/30 seconds intervals at 4.0 mph and 7.0 to 8.0 mph, or a speed that makes you feel somewhat uncomfortable. Do 45 minutes of intervals for a total of 60 minutes including the warm-up.

Making the Cut: Real People, Real Results

Name: Stevland Turner
Age: 38
Location: Burbank, California
Occupation: Self-employed
Height: 6'0"
Starting weight: 272 pounds
Ending weight: 236.2 pounds

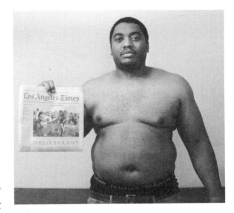

I've wanted to lose weight for about 12 years. I've tried other diets and exercise plans before, but I didn't stay motivated because I didn't get results fast enough. I decided to make a change in my life, and Obi is an example of where I want to be fitness-wise in the long run, so I decided to try the Cut program.

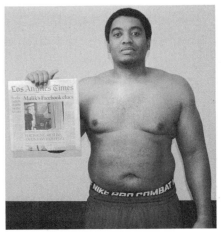

I thought the program might turn out to be the same as other diets, but I started to see a difference in my body about three weeks in. The Cut program gave me a plan to follow so I didn't feel like I was out there without a rudder. Having set things to do— the diet and the workouts—is important with a program like this.

Now that I've finished the 12 weeks, I feel great and like I'm definitely on the road to getting to the body that I want. I'd tell someone considering The Cut to do it. Stick with it. Twelve weeks isn't that long a time, and three months are going to pass anyway!

> The Cut program gave me a plan to follow so I didn't feel like I was out there without a rudder. Having set things to do—the diet and the workouts—is important with a program like this.

8 Boot Camp Cardio Exercises

Most people do too much of the wrong kind of cardio exercise. Look, you're not going to sculpt your body or get Cut while strolling on the treadmill or mindlessly pedaling an elliptical trainer. To shed fat and get shredded, the key is intensity. The boot camp moves like the ones in this chapter can be done anywhere—in your living room or at the gym—and will definitely get (and keep!) your heart rate up.

You should perform each of these moves for 30 to 45 seconds at a time; that's 1 set. If you're new to working out and can only do a move for less time than that, just gradually work up to that 30- to 45-second mark and eventually aim to do 3 to 4 sets, depending on the workout. You'll rest for about a minute between sets. (If you're very fit, you can cut that rest time to 30 to 45 seconds.) Each of these moves is a cardio exercise that will get your heart pumping and burn tons of calories while you're performing it.

MOUNTAIN CLIMBER

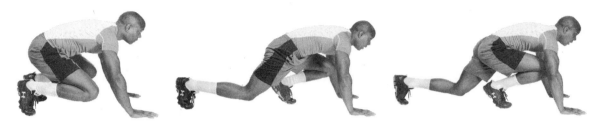

This exercise works the core, glutes, quads, and hamstrings.

Place your hands on the floor, shoulder-width apart, with your feet under your hips. Pull your right knee toward your chest and then do the same with your left leg as you step your right foot back (as if you were "climbing" the floor). Continue to alternate legs as you perform the exercise. Do for 30 to 45 seconds.

JUMPING JACK

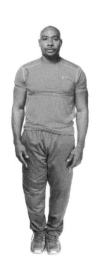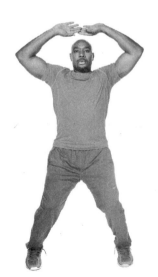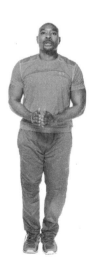

This plyometric, or jumping, move is a simple but challenging cardio exercise.

Stand with your feet together, knees slightly bent, arms at your sides. Jump your legs apart, landing on the balls of your feet, while simultaneously bringing your hands up over your head; then bring your legs back under your hips while you bring your arms back down to your sides. Do for 30 to 45 seconds.

From Obi:

Exercise used to be considered optional by doctors. Now doctors know that regular exercise promotes longevity and reduces the risk of developing many common diseases. No wonder so many physicians are prescribing it for their patients!

BURPEE

This challenging cardio exercise includes a plyometric component and will get you in great shape.

Stand with your feet shoulder-distance apart and bend your knees to perform a squat, pushing your butt back and down as you keep your knees behind your toes. As you do so, put your hands on the ground and jump your feet back, as if you're going to perform a push-up. Immediately jump your feet back under your shoulders and leap up, reaching your arms toward the ceiling. Do for 30 to 45 seconds. (See next page.)

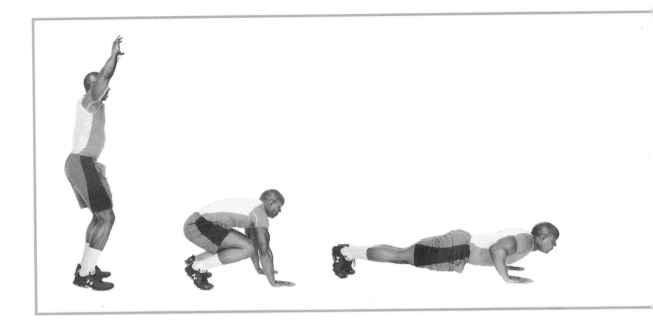

SKI JUMP

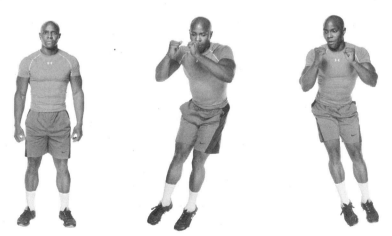

This cardio exercise includes a plyometric component.

Stand with your feet shoulder-distance apart, knees slightly bent. With your arms bent and by your sides (as if you were holding ski poles), jump from right side to left side, keeping your legs parallel and slightly closer than shoulder-distance apart, using your arms for balance. Jump as far as you can and focus on landing as lightly as possible. Do for 30 to 45 seconds.

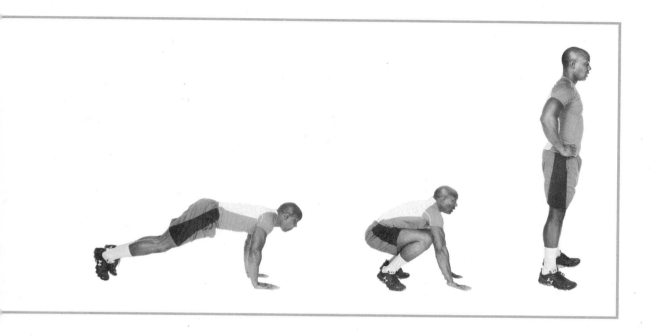

HIGH KNEE

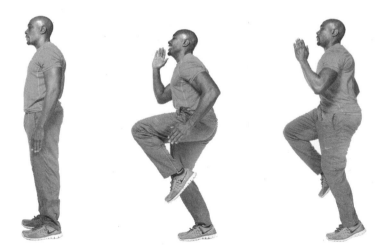

This cardio exercise also engages your abs and core.

Stand with your feet shoulder-width apart, arms at your sides with your elbows bent. Lift each knee one at a time high enough so that your thighs are parallel to the ground and run fast in place, landing softly on the balls of your feet. Do for 30 to 45 seconds.

QUICK FEET

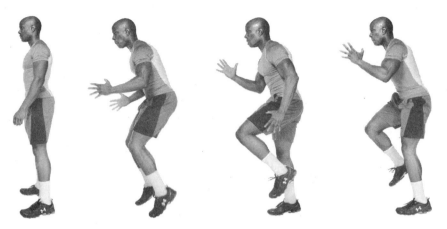

This cardio exercise improves your endurance and agility.

Stand with your feet shoulder-width apart, arms bent and at your sides, weight on the balls of your feet. Run in place, moving as quickly as possible and landing as lightly as you can (as if you were stepping on eggshells). Do for 30 to 45 seconds.

SQUAT UPPERCUT

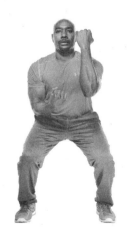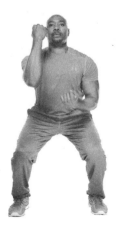

This cardio exercise works the quads, hamstrings, glutes, calves, and core.

Stand with your feet shoulder-width apart and your knees bent, keeping your knees behind your toes, as if you were going to sit in a chair behind you. Your knees should make 90-degree angles. As you hold that position with your back straight, make a fist with your left hand and punch upward as if you were going to punch someone under his chin. This is an uppercut. Repeat, making a fist and punching upward with your right arm. Continue to hold the static squat while you make uppercuts with each arm. Do for 30 to 45 seconds.

RUN AROUND THE TOWEL

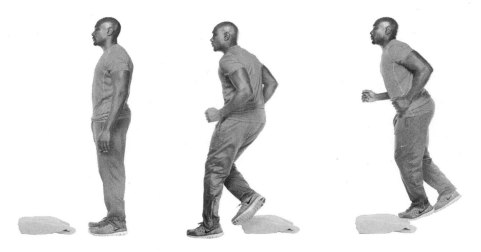

This cardio exercise gets your heart rate up quickly.

Place a towel flat on the ground and run around it in a circle, staying on the balls of your feet. Run in a circle, landing as lightly as you can, using your arms at your sides for balance. Do for 30 to 45 seconds.

SUICIDE

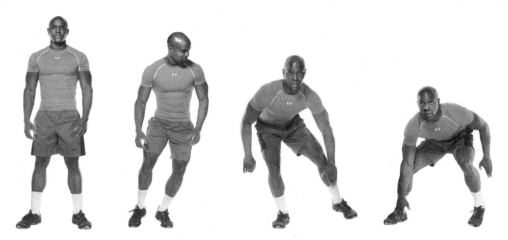

This cardio exercise works the glutes, quads, hamstrings, and calves. It's challenging, so pace yourself during the first few sets.

Place a marker or cone 5 to 7 feet away from you. Run as fast as you can from your starting point to the marker or cone; touch the marker; and then run backward to your starting position. Do for 30 to 45 seconds.

SWITCH FEET

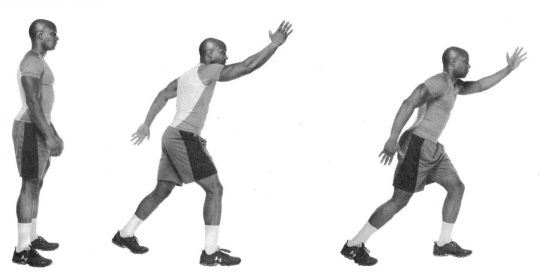

This cardio exercise includes a plyometric component and builds endurance.
Stand with your feet shoulder-distance apart, arms at your sides. Step your right foot forward and your left foot back and then jump your left foot forward and right foot back, swinging opposite arms for momentum and balance. Move your feet as quickly as you can while landing softly. Do for 30 to 45 seconds.

From Morris:

I actually love doing basketball jump shots because they help my vertical jump on the court, too.

BASKETBALL JUMP SHOT

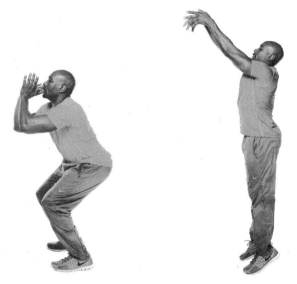

This is a plyometric and cardio move that uses your entire body, including your core.
Stand with your feet shoulder-distance apart and bend your knees, pushing your bottom back and down and keeping your knees behind your toes. Keep your hands in front of you (as if you're holding a basketball). Explode up from this position as if you were making a jump shot; land with your legs bent and repeat. Do for 30 to 45 seconds.

9 Leg Exercises

Your legs contain the largest muscles in your body, and training them the right way will help you expend more calories and burn more fat overall. If you're a woman and are concerned that training your legs will bulk them up, don't worry. Adding muscle will give your legs definition and tone and even reduce the look of cellulite, so don't fear the exercises in this chapter! While sometimes men overlook training their legs, focusing on their upper bodies, adding muscle to your legs will rev your metabolism and give you a stronger, more balanced physique.

Leg exercises that require a minimum of equipment and can be done at home are listed first. Leg exercises that use gym equipment appear later in the chapter.

A Word About Weights

Exercising at home? Many of the strength exercises in the following chapters require no equipment; you'll need dumbbells for others. If you don't own dumbbells already, consider purchasing several pairs you can keep and use at home. Men might start with 15- to 20-pound weights while women can choose lighter ones like 5 to 10 pounds.

If you don't want to spend the money, you can use household items for the moves. A gallon jug of water or milk, canned goods, and even containers of dishwashing detergent can serve as added resistance. Once you are regularly lifting weights of more than 5 to 10 pounds, however, we suggest investing in a set or two of dumbbells—or working out at a gym where you'll have access to them.

HOME LEG EXERCISES

BODY-WEIGHT SQUAT

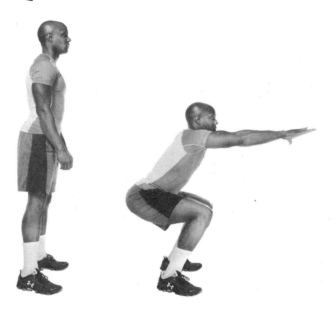

Squats work the glutes, hamstrings, quads, calves, and even abs: As you perform the exercise, your core is naturally engaged.

Start with your feet shoulder-width apart, toes pointing out slightly to engage your glutes. You can keep your arms at your sides, or hold them out in front of you for balance. Keeping your back straight with your weight in your heels, bend your knees until they make 90-degree angles—as if you were going to sit in a chair behind you. Inhale as you bend your knees, and keep them behind your toes. When you reach 90 degrees, pause briefly and then exhale as you return to your original position. (If you have knee pain that prevents you from squatting that deeply, squat as low as is comfortable.)

Aim for 15 to 20 reps for 3 to 4 sets, resting for 1 minute between sets. To increase the challenge, hold dumbbells at your sides.

WALL SIT

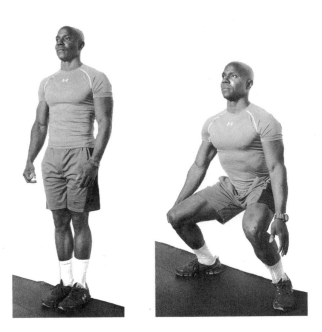

This exercise targets the quadriceps, hamstrings, calves, and abs. If you have knee issues, you needn't lower yourself to make 90-degree angles with your knees—stop before you feel any discomfort. You'll still get benefits from holding the position.

Stand with your back against a wall, and place your feet shoulder-distance apart. Keeping your abs engaged, with your arms at your sides, slide your body down the wall until your knees are bent; hold the position for at least 30 seconds and up to 60 seconds if you really want to challenge yourself, breathing normally before returning to your starting position. (If you can't hold the position for 30 seconds, just hold for as long as you can and then return to the starting position.)

The 30- to 60-second hold counts as 1 set; aim for 3 to 4 sets. Rest for 1 minute between sets.

LUNGE

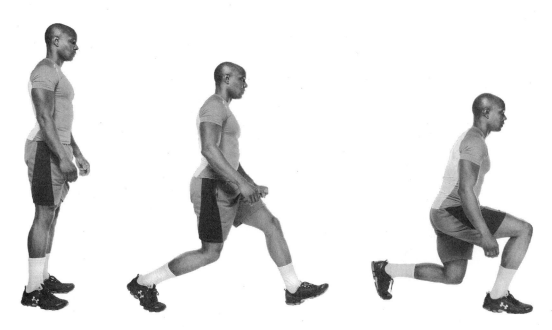

This exercise works the quadriceps, glutes, inner thighs, hamstrings, and calves.

Stand with your feet shoulder-distance apart and inhale as you step far enough forward with your right foot so that both knees will make 90-degree angles as you lower your left knee toward the ground. Keep your chest up and your abs engaged. Pause briefly and exhale as you step your right foot back to the starting position. Repeat, stepping forward with your left foot. That's 1 rep.

Aim for 12 to 15 reps for 3 to 4 sets. Rest for 1 minute between sets. To make the move more challenging, hold dumbbells at your sides.

BODY-WEIGHT CALF RAISE

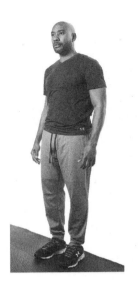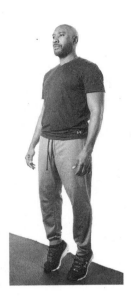

This exercise targets the calf muscles.

Stand with your feet shoulder-distance apart with your arms at your sides. Keeping your legs straight, exhale as you slowly lift your heels off the ground to bring your weight onto the balls of your feet and then return to the starting position as you inhale.

Your calf muscles are relatively small compared with the rest of your leg muscles, so you'll do more repetitions of this exercise—aim for 3 to 4 sets of 25 to 30 reps each. Rest for 1 minute between sets. To increase the challenge, hold dumbbells at your sides.

GYM LEG EXERCISES

The following exercises require equipment you'll find at your gym or health club. We've given detailed instructions about how to perform each move, but don't hesitate to ask a staff member or employee if you have any questions about how to use the equipment. Most weight-lifting machines must be adjusted to fit your body—by raising or lowering a seat, for example—for safe use. A staff member can also help you determine the appropriate weight to lift. In general, the amount of weight you lift should be 50 to 70 percent of your 1-rep maximum weight, or the highest amount of weight you can lift one time.

LEG PRESS
(uses leg press machine)

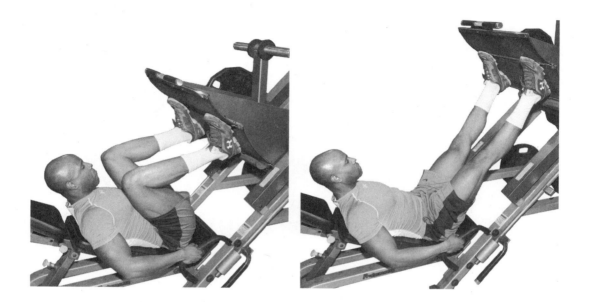

This exercise targets the quads, hamstrings, and calves.

Place your feet on the leg press platform slightly wider than shoulder-width apart, with your back against the machine's pad, hands at your sides holding the handles, knees bent at 90-degree angles. Exhale as you contract your quads (the muscles in the front of your thighs) and extend your legs until they're straight with soft knees (without locking your knees); pause briefly and then return to your original position as you inhale.

Warm up with a light weight for your first set, and gradually increase the weight with each set.

Aim for 12 to 15 repetitions for 3 to 4 sets.

LEG EXTENSION
(uses leg extension machine)

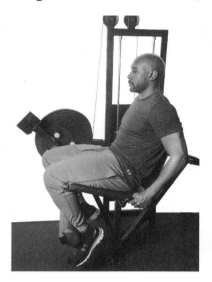 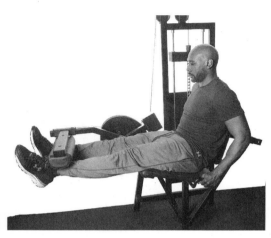

This exercise targets the quads.

Sit on the leg extension machine with your back against the seat, roller pads against the fronts of your shins, and your knees lined up with the fulcrum of the machine. Hold the handles of the machine and exhale as you extend your legs until they're straight without locking your knees; pause briefly and inhale as you return to your original position. Warm up using a light weight for your first set and gradually increase the weight with each set.

Aim for 12 to 15 reps for 3 to 4 sets.

From Morris:

Legs are probably my hardest body part to train. I think I train them the most, but they're still my weakest body part. I know I'm really hitting them right if I get really sore afterward.

CALF RAISE ON LEG PRESS MACHINE
(uses leg press machine)

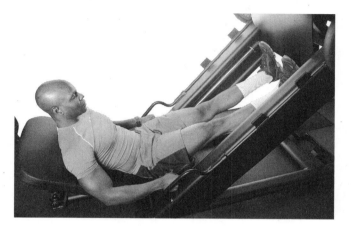

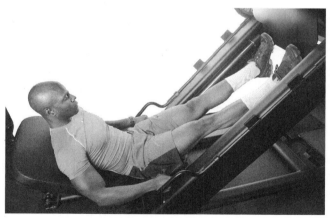

This exercise targets the calf muscles.

Place your feet on the leg press platform slightly wider than shoulder-width apart, with your back against the machine's pad, hands at your sides holding the handles, knees bent at 90-degree angles. Exhale as you contract your quads (the muscles in the front of your thighs) and extend your legs until they're straight with soft knees (without locking your knees). Lift your heels to bring your weight onto the balls of your feet; pause briefly and lower your heels without letting them touch the ground. That's 1 rep.

Aim for 20 to 25 reps for 3 to 4 sets.

SMITH MACHINE SQUAT
(uses Smith machine)

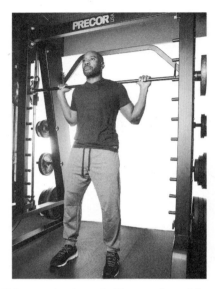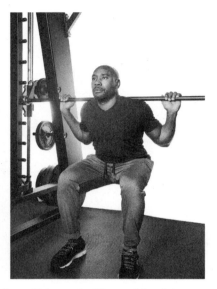

This exercise targets the quads and hamstrings. Using a Smith machine lets you use more weight without worrying about balance issues, so intermediate and advanced exercisers may want to use a Smith machine to do squats so they can lift more weight.

Start with your feet shoulder-width apart, toes pointed out slightly to engage your glutes, shoulders under the padded bar, legs slightly bent. Keeping your weight in your heels, bend your knees until they make 90-degree angles. Inhale as you bend your knees, and keep them behind your toes. When your knees reach 90 degrees, pause briefly and then exhale as you return to your original position. The deeper you squat, the more you'll feel this exercise in your hamstrings.

Aim for 10 to 12 reps for 3 to 4 sets.

PRONE LEG CURL
(uses prone leg curl machine)

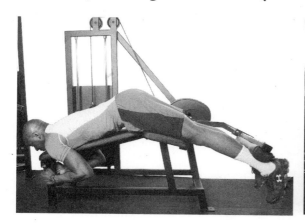 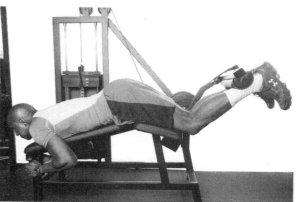

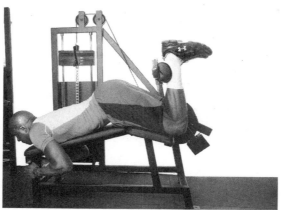

This exercise works the hamstrings and butt.

Lie flat on the leg curl machine on your stomach, legs extended and the pad positioned on the backs of your ankles, holding the handles on either side of the machine. Keep your thighs pressed against the machine as you contract your hamstrings to pull the pad toward your butt; pause briefly and return to your original position.

Aim for 12 to 15 reps for 3 to 4 sets.

10 Chest Exercises

What does a strong chest do for you? If you're a guy, it makes you look younger and more powerful. If you're a woman, a stronger chest gives your breasts more support, making you look—yup, you guessed it—younger, and slimmer, too, as your waist looks smaller in comparison.

There are several primary exercises that target your chest muscles—namely push-ups, chest presses, and chest flies. Changing how you perform the exercises—by doing chest presses on an incline bench instead of a flat one, for example—will target different parts of your chest for a balanced, symmetrical look. You'll find the home exercises first, followed by the gym exercises.

HOME CHEST EXERCISES

PUSH-UP

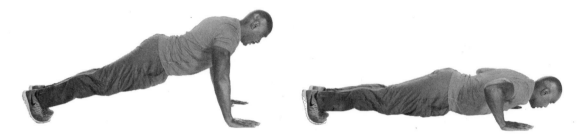

This exercise targets the chest, shoulders, and triceps.

Lie facedown with your hands just outside your shoulders. Engage your abs and push your body up so that you're on your hands and toes, keeping your body in a straight line. Inhale as you bend your elbows to the sides to lower your chest until it touches the ground; pause briefly and then exhale to push yourself back to the starting position. Keep your back straight during the exercise. Do 10 to 12 reps for 3 to 4 sets. Rest for 1 minute between sets.

MODIFIED PUSH-UP

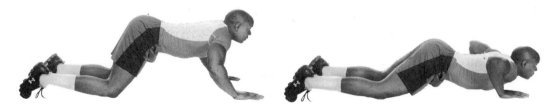

Not everyone can do regular push-ups. Beginning exercisers and those who are still building upper-body strength should start with modified push-ups. This exercise targets the chest, shoulders, and triceps.

Lie facedown with your hands under your shoulders. Engage your abs and push your body up so that you're on your hands and knees. Keeping your body in a straight line, inhale as you bend your elbows to lower your chest until it nearly touches the ground; pause briefly and then exhale to push yourself back to the starting position. Keep your back straight during the exercise. Do 10 to 12 reps for 3 to 4 sets. Rest for 1 minute between sets.

INCLINE PUSH-UP
(using bench or box)

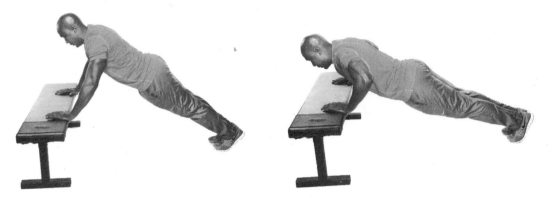

This exercise targets the chest, shoulders, and triceps; it works the upper chest more than traditional push-ups.

Place your hands shoulder-distance apart on the edge of a weight bench, sturdy coffee table, or low sofa. Engage your abs so that you're in push-up position with your upper body higher than your feet. Inhale as you lower your body until your elbows make 90-degree angles; exhale as you push yourself back up to the starting position. Keep your back straight during the exercise. Do 10 to 12 reps for 3 to 4 sets. Rest for 1 minute between sets.

From Morris:

I don't do much bench-pressing these days! But just about every day, I do push-ups to work my chest and triceps. I get a good pump from that, and my chest stays pretty strong.

GYM CHEST EXERCISES

CHEST PRESS
(uses weight bench)

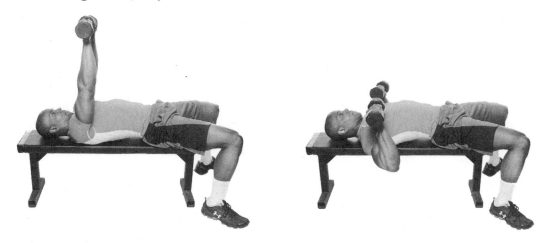

This exercise targets the chest, shoulders, and triceps.

    Lie on the bench on your back, holding dumbbells in both hands at chest level, elbows bent at 90-degree angles (like a football goalpost). Exhale as you press the dumbbells toward the ceiling; inhale as you bring the dumbbells back to your starting position. Do 10 to 12 reps for 3 to 4 sets.

INCLINE CHEST PRESS
(uses incline weight bench)

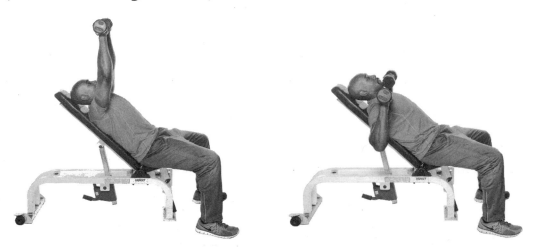

This exercise targets the upper chest, shoulders, and triceps.

Lie on an incline bench, holding dumbbells in both hands at chest level, elbows bent at 90-degree angles (like a football goalpost). Exhale as you press the dumbbells toward the ceiling; inhale as you bring the dumbbells back to the starting position. Do 10 to 12 reps for 3 to 4 sets.

UPRIGHT FLY
(uses butterfly chest machine)

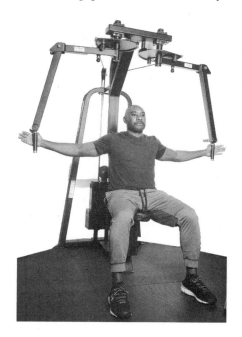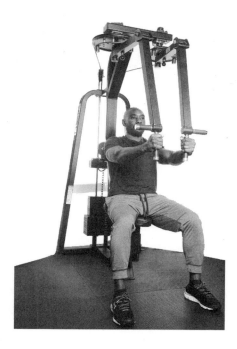

This exercise targets the chest.

Sit on the machine with your back against the pad, and grasp the handles with your arms parallel to the floor. Squeeze your chest as you exhale and pull the handles together in front of your chest; pause briefly and inhale as you return your arms to the starting position. Do 10 to 12 reps for 3 or 4 sets.

11 | Back Exercises

When people lift weights, they often focus on the muscles they see in the mirror—their chests, shoulders, arms, legs, and, of course, abs! While you don't see your back when you look in the mirror, you want to make sure you train it as intensely as your "mirror" muscles. Training your back along with the front of your body will make you look symmetrical and avoid any muscular imbalances. Your back, chest, and legs contain the biggest muscle groups, so adding muscle to your back will also boost your metabolism.

If you're a man, you're probably aiming for a more V-taper to your upper body; these exercises will help you attain that. Women will get the same results to a lesser degree—a strong back makes you look sleek and toned.

Note that because training your back requires that you pull something toward you, your home exercise options are somewhat limited. The bent-over row is the classic home exercise and is the most efficient dumbbell exercise to strengthen your back, but if you want more options, you'll want to try the moves that use gym equipment.

HOME BACK EXERCISE

BENT-OVER ROW

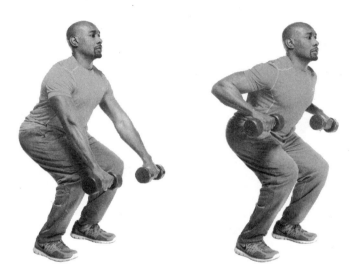

This exercise targets the back.

Stand with your feet shoulder-distance apart and hinge forward at the waist. Your knees will be slightly bent; keep your abs engaged and hold dumbbells in both hands with your arms straight. Exhale as you bend your arms to "row" your hands toward your hips, making 90-degree angles with your elbows; pause briefly before returning to your original position.

Do 12 to 15 reps for 3 to 4 sets.

From Morris:

The back is probably the body part I work out the least. Before working out with Obi, I hadn't hit my back in ages. Now I've got in my head that I need to work my back—and I'm a lot stronger. I went from being able to only do a few pull-ups at a time to doing 4 sets of 12 pull-ups!

GYM BACK EXERCISES

PULL-UP
(uses pull-up bar)

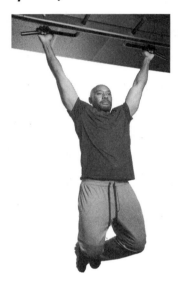 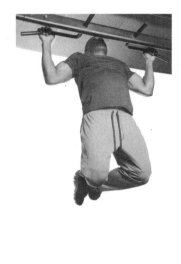

This exercise targets the back and arms. This is a challenging move that most women and many men cannot perform. Unless you're used to doing push-ups, you should use the weight-assisted pull-up machine.

Grab a pull-up bar with your palms shoulder-width apart. Keeping your abs engaged, exhale as you pull your body up with your arms until your chin passes the bar; pause briefly and then lower your body to the starting position as you inhale.

Do 10 to 12 reps for 3 to 4 sets.

LAT PULL-DOWN
(uses lat pull-down machine)

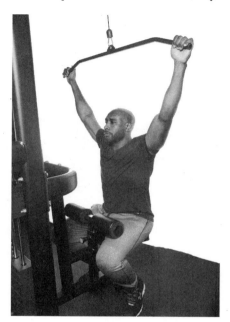 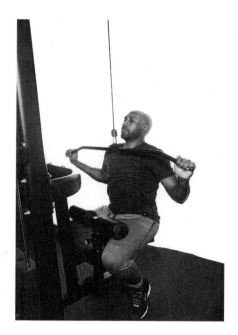

This exercise targets the back and arms.

Sit on the seat of the machine and adjust the thigh pads so that your quads, or thighs, are comfortable. Grab the handle of the pull-down bar with a wide overhand grip. Keeping your shoulders retracted, exhale as you pull the bar down to your chest; pause briefly and then inhale as you return to your starting position. Keep your back straight and your abs engaged during the exercise.

Do 10 to 12 reps for 3 to 4 sets.

SEATED LOW ROW
(uses low pulley machine)

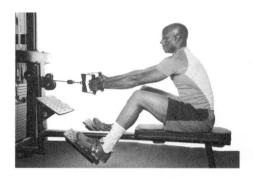 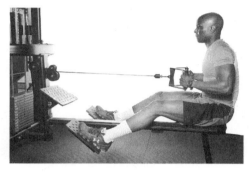

This exercise targets the back.

Adjust the pulley machine so that it's at a low setting, and use a V-bar attachment. Sit on the machine with your feet on the platform, knees slightly bent, and grasp the V-bar in your hands, with your back slightly arched. Engage your abs and exhale as you pull the V-bar toward your abs; pause briefly and inhale as you return to the starting position.

Do 10 to 12 reps for 3 to 4 sets.

T-BAR ROW
(uses cable machine and T-bar attachment)

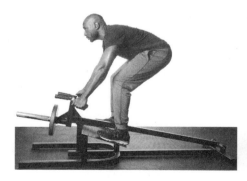 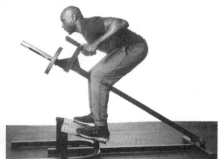

This exercise targets the back.

Stand over the T-bar with your feet under your hips, and grab the T-bar with both hands. Engage your abs, keep your shoulders retracted, and exhale as you pull the T-bar toward your chest; pause briefly and then lower the T-bar back toward the ground as you inhale.

Do 10 to 12 reps for 3 to 4 sets.

12 Arm Exercises

Toned arms tell the world something—that you're fit and strong. We know guys—including us—love to show off impressive guns. Training your arms the right way will build both your biceps (the muscles in the front of your arms) and your triceps (the muscles in the back of your arms) to give you more size and definition.

If you're a woman, you may not want bigger arms, but you probably would love to have sleeker ones! The exercises in this chapter will help you tone the backs of your arms (a notorious problem area!) and give you a more sculpted, feminine look. You'll find the home exercises first, followed by those to do at the gym.

Making the Cut: Real People, Real Results

Name: Renee Carter
Age: 45
Location: Atlanta, Georgia
Occupation: Paralegal
Height: 5'8"
Starting weight: 286 pounds
Ending weight: 266 pounds

My weight has been a constant battle since I had children. (I have a 21-year-old son and 18-year-old twin girls.) I needed to lose weight desperately, and I needed some help.

I felt overweight and sluggish when I started The Cut. I stayed on the plan by preparing my meals in advance, and the gym is right around the corner from my job, which made it easier. I did have to change my mind-set to make working out part of my regular routine—it's a requirement, not a request! My weight won't lose itself—if I could send someone to the gym for me, I would, but I can't! So I had to roll with the punches.

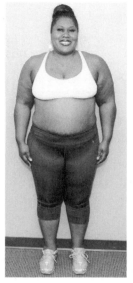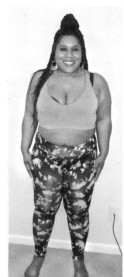

I started to notice a difference in my body about six to eight weeks in. I liked the weight-lifting part and the cardio—the running has opened up another door for me. I haven't been able to run in a long time, and now I'm trying to build myself up to run a mile and eventually do a 5K race.

The Cut has given me back my drive for working out…and I have more energy and my blood pressure is back down.

> I did have to change my mind-set to make working out part of my regular routine—it's a requirement, not a request! My weight won't lose itself.

HOME ARM EXERCISES

DIP

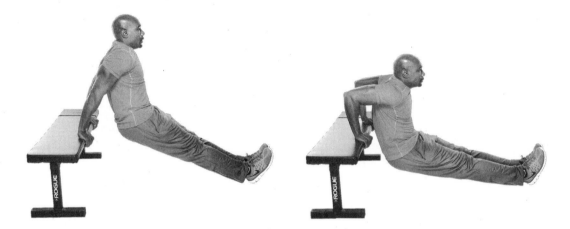

This exercise targets the triceps and shoulders.

Sit on a chair (or weight bench) with your hands on the edge, shoulder-width apart, with your legs bent in front of you. (The farther your feet are from you, the more challenging this exercise is. As you get stronger, you can straighten your legs and place your feet farther from the chair.) Straighten your arms to lift your butt off the chair and inhale as you dip your body down by bending your arms until your elbows make 90-degree angles. Your body should stay close to the chair; your butt will brush the bench. Exhale as you push back up to your starting position.

Do 10 to 12 reps for 3 or 4 sets.

TRICEPS KICKBACK

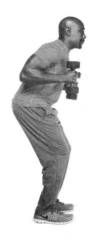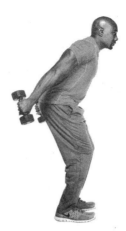

This exercise targets the triceps.

Stand with your feet shoulder-distance apart and hinge from the hips, holding dumbbells at your sides with your elbows bent. Keep your upper arms close to your body and exhale as you straighten your arms to bring the dumbbells above your hips; pause briefly and return to the starting position, stopping when your elbows make 90-degree angles.

Do 10 to 12 reps for 3 to 4 sets.

TRICEPS PUSH-UP

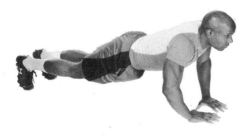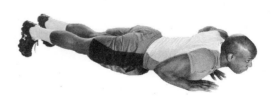

This exercise targets the triceps, upper chest, and shoulders.

Lie facedown with your hands next to your shoulders. Engage your abs and push your body up so that you're on your hands and toes; inhale as you bend your elbows to lower your chest until it touches the ground; pause briefly and then exhale to push yourself back to the starting position. (This exercise is identical to a regular push-up but the hand position puts the emphasis on the triceps muscles.) Keep your back straight during the exercise.

Do 10 to 12 reps for 3 to 4 sets.

From Morris:

I listen to music when I work out all the time. I'll like hip-hop and straight R&B and slow songs, depending on what my mood is. A lot of the time, I listen to news and interviews to stay on top of what people are doing and saying. It makes training more fun.

BICEPS CURL

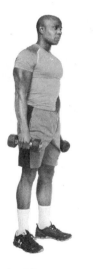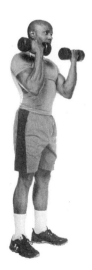

This exercise targets the biceps.

Stand with your feet shoulder-distance apart, holding dumbbells at your sides. Exhale as you bend your elbows to bring the dumbbells up to your shoulders; inhale as you lower the dumbbells back to the starting position. Make sure to bring the dumbbells all the way down with each repetition to work your entire biceps muscle, and keep your elbows soft (don't lock them) at the bottom of the rep. Keep your arms close to your body and avoid swinging your body or using momentum to lift the dumbbells.

Do 10 to 12 reps for 3 to 4 sets.

GYM ARM EXERCISES

TRICEPS PUSH-DOWN
(uses cable machine with triceps bar)

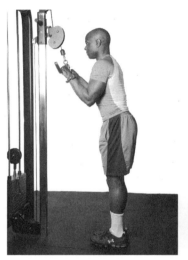 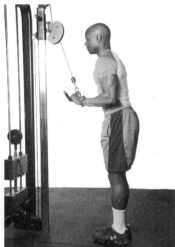 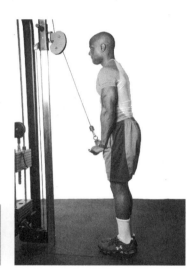

This exercise targets the triceps.

Stand at the cable machine and pull the triceps bar down to your belly with your elbows bent to 90-degree angles; exhale as you extend your arms to push the bar down to your thighs, keeping your arms close to your body. Inhale as you let the bar come back to the starting position.

Do 10 to 12 reps for 3 to 4 sets.

From Obi:

When training your triceps, make sure to keep your arms close to your body. This helps isolate your triceps muscles for better results.

CABLE BICEPS CURL
(uses cable machine)

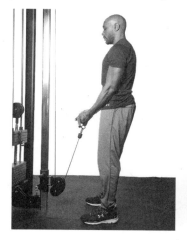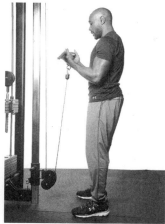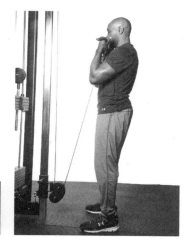

This exercise targets the biceps.

Stand at the cable machine and hold the cable bar at thigh level with an underhand grip, hands shoulder-distance apart. Keep your arms close to your body and exhale as you bend your arms to bring the bar up to your shoulders; inhale as you lower the bar back to your thighs.

Do 10 to 12 reps for 3 to 4 sets.

PREACHER CURL
(uses preacher curl bench)

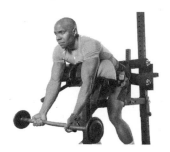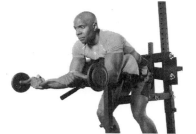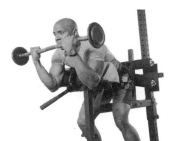

This exercise targets the biceps.

Sit on the preacher curl bench with dumbbells or an EZ bar in your hands and place your arms on top of the pad with your palms facing up; your arms will be at a 90-degree angle. Inhale as you lower the dumbbells until your arms are fully stretched out; exhale as you curl the dumbbells back to your starting position.

Do 10 to 12 reps for 3 to 4 sets.

SEATED HAMMER CURL

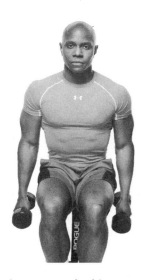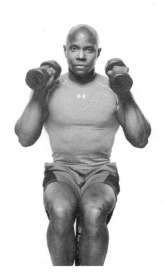

This exercise targets the biceps.

Sit on the edge of a weight bench with your feet shoulder-distance apart on the ground, holding dumbbells at your sides with your palms facing your body. Keeping your hands in the same position and your elbows close to your body, exhale as you curl the dumbbells up to your shoulders; inhale as you lower the dumbbells back to the starting position.

Do 10 to 12 reps for 3 to 4 sets.

13 Shoulder Exercises

Shoulders are sometimes an afterthought when it comes to lifting weights, but strong shoulders make you look taller and improve your posture. Sculpted shoulders look great on women of any age, and guys often strive to develop eye-popping shoulders that enhance their chest and arms.

When you train your chest doing exercises like push-ups and chest presses, your shoulders get a little work, too. They also stabilize you during other exercises like triceps push-downs. The exercises in this chapter, however, specifically target your shoulder muscles. You'll find home exercises listed first, followed by gym exercises.

HOME SHOULDER EXERCISES

SHOULDER PRESS

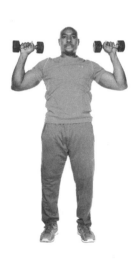 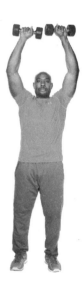

This exercise targets the shoulders.

Stand with your feet shoulder-distance apart, holding dumbbells just above your shoulders with your elbows bent toward your torso and palms facing up. Engage your abs and exhale as you press the dumbbells up over your head until your arms are straight; inhale as you lower them back to the starting position.

Do 10 to 12 reps for 3 to 4 sets.

LATERAL RAISE

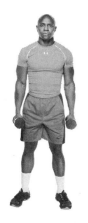
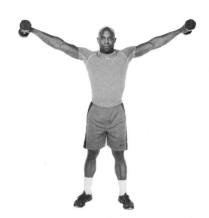

This exercise targets the mid-shoulders.

Stand with your feet shoulder-distance apart, holding dumbbells at your sides, palms facing your body. Your arms should be straight, but your elbows remain soft, not locked. Exhale as you raise your arms to just above shoulder height; inhale as you lower the dumbbells to your sides.

Do 10 to 12 reps for 3 to 4 sets.

UPRIGHT ROW

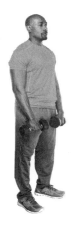
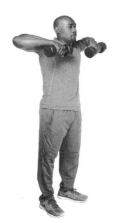

This exercise targets the shoulders.

Stand with your feet shoulder-distance apart, holding dumbbells in front of your thighs, palms facing your thighs. Bend your arms to "row" the dumbbells up to your chest as you exhale (your elbows will move up and away from your body); inhale as you lower the dumbbells to the starting position.

Do 10 to 12 reps for 3 to 4 sets.

FRONT RAISE

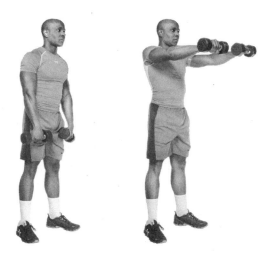

This exercise targets the front of the shoulders.

Stand with your feet shoulder-distance apart, holding dumbbells in front of your thighs, palms facing your thighs. Keeping your arms straight, exhale as you raise the dumbbells to shoulder height; inhale as you lower the dumbbells to the starting position.

Do 10 to 12 reps for 3 to 4 sets.

SHOULDER SHRUG

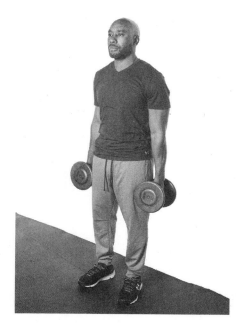 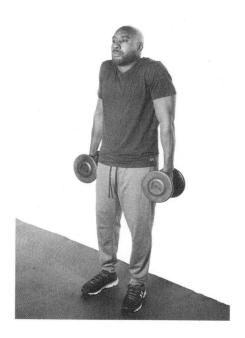

This exercise targets the shoulders.

Stand with your feet hip-distance apart, holding dumbbells in front of your thighs, palms facing your thighs. Keeping your arms straight, exhale as you slowly shrug your shoulders to lift the dumbbells up a few inches; inhale as you return to original position.

Do 10 to 12 reps for 3 to 4 sets.

Making the Cut: Real People, Real Results

Name: Oluwole Awosika
Age: 33
Location: Kensington, Maryland
Occupation: Neurologist/scientist
Height: 5'8"
Starting weight: 235.2 pounds
Ending weight: 214 pounds

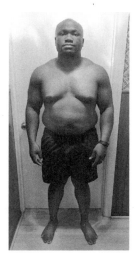

When I started The Cut, I was a bit hungry the first couple of days; then I became less hungry and in fact had to constantly remind myself to eat the between-meal snacks. Also, I started to feel more and more energetic. I found it challenging to keep a slow pace during the recovery intervals of my interval training because I felt so pumped and faster than I used to be!

I noticed a change in how I felt within the first four days of starting the program. I feel energized and have a better appreciation for eating a well-balanced diet. Now I feel equipped with the knowledge needed to not only lose weight, but maintain a healthy weight and lifestyle. For this I am eternally grateful.

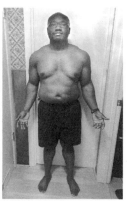

Getting in great shape required work and discipline. Hence, the discipline I learned from doing this program not only helped me achieve my weight loss and fitness goals but also transcended into other aspects of my life, such as improving my planning and organizational skills—which also led to greater efficiency at work.

> I noticed a change in how I felt within the first four days of starting the program. I feel energized and have a better appreciation for eating a well-balanced diet.

GYM SHOULDER EXERCISES

SEATED SHOULDER PRESS
(uses weight bench)

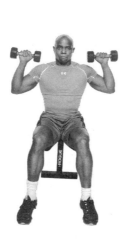
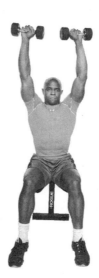

This exercise targets the shoulders.

Sit on a weight bench with your feet shoulder-distance apart, holding dumbbells just above your shoulders with your elbows bent by your torso and your palms facing up. Engage your abs and exhale as you press the dumbbells up over your head until your arms are straight; inhale as you lower them back to your starting position.

Do 10 to 12 reps for 3 to 4 sets.

SEATED SIDE RAISE

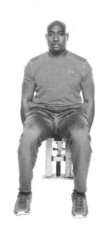
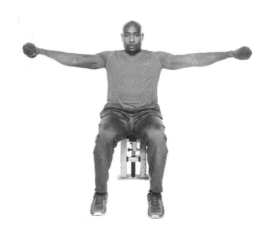

This exercise targets the mid-shoulders.

Sit on a bench with your feet under your hips, holding dumbbells at your sides, palms facing your body. Exhale as you raise your arms to shoulder height; inhale as you lower the dumbbells to your sides.

Do 10 to 12 reps for 3 to 4 sets.

14 Ab Exercises

Is there any body part more sought after than a flat, sexy stomach if you're a woman or washboard, shredded abs if you're a guy? In chapter 2 you learned that if you want to see your abs, you've got to get your body fat down—that will bring those abs out of hibernation!

How do you do that? By using a combination of diet, cardio, and circuit training to torch fat. Doing a variety of different ab exercises will help you strengthen and build these muscles so that when that fat has melted away, you'll be proud to show them off.

This chapter includes effective ab exercises you can do at home (requiring no equipment) or using gym equipment. Each is designed to help you build that sexy, lean midsection you've always wanted. (Note that different exercises have different rep counts or seconds to hold, depending on the move.)

Making the Cut: Real People, Real Results

Name: Osborn H. "Tiger" Christon Jr.
Age: 47
Location: McKinney, Texas
Occupation: Insurance claim specialist
Height: 6'4"
Starting weight: 278.8 pounds
Ending weight: 248.6 pounds

I have been struggling with my weight and physical fitness since I completed my collegiate football career in 1991. I've tried other diets and exercise plans but

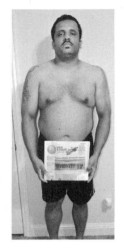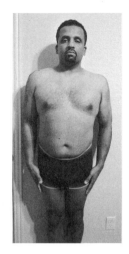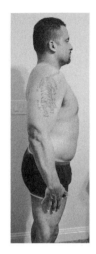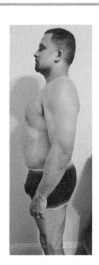

didn't see immediate results. I was tired of past failures and made up my mind that I was going to do my best and complete The Cut.

I'm married with three children and work full-time; my challenge was time. How could I balance my responsibilities at work and at home in order to complete this program? My wife and children have been very supportive, which made it easier for me. My wife adjusted her daily schedule, which freed up time to accommodate my workout schedule. She also took on some of my responsibilities at home and with my children, which inspired me to accomplish my goals.

My children noticed my transformation and continuously encouraged me to stay on course. In fact, halfway through the program, my family started eating the Cut dinners. They have changed some of their eating habits since I started the program and are making better, healthier choices. Both my wife and children are more interested in exercising and going to the gym with Dad.

After starting the Cut program, I immediately saw a difference in my body! Within the first 10 days, I lost 9 pounds and felt a lot stronger. I felt my "muscle memory" coming back, which increased every week. This was also a big motivator for me not to give up.

After 12 weeks, I feel totally transformed! I feel healthier and more energetic. My family and friends have noticed the change in me both physically and mentally. Eating healthy is now a habit for me, and I'm much more conscious of my food choices.

The Cut has been a lifestyle change for me. I'm committed to continue the principles I've learned throughout this program. I have proven to myself that with discipline and hard work, I can accomplish any goals I set for myself.

I would definitely recommend this program to anyone who wants to lose weight and get physically fit the natural way…hard work and dedication pay off in the long run!

After 12 weeks, I feel totally transformed! I feel healthier and more energetic. My family and friends have noticed the change in me both physically and mentally.

HOME AB EXERCISES

PLANK

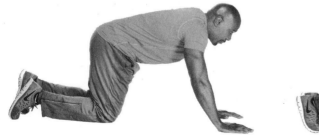 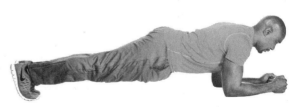

This exercise targets both the upper and lower abs, including obliques.

Lie facedown with your forearms on the floor, palms down, feet under your hips. Push up onto your toes and forearms, engaging your core to keep your body in a straight line without letting your hips stick up or sag. Keep your shoulders positioned over your forearms, and breathe normally while you keep your body straight; hold for 30 to 45 seconds for 3 to 4 sets.

Making the Cut: Real People, Real Results

Name: Donna Eggleston
Age: 56
Location: Chicago, Illinois
Occupation: Social worker
Height: 5'9"
Starting weight: 229.8 pounds
Ending weight: 207.2 pounds

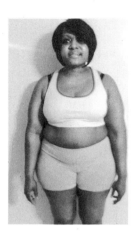

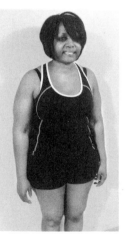

In addition to wanting to lose weight, I have some joint issues, but I believed that The Cut would work for me. And it did! I felt a difference in my body after the first week—I lost 4 pounds! That definitely increased my confidence level and kept my motivation going.

The overall program is very challenging—you definitely have to have razor focus to do it. My biggest challenges were the planks, push-ups, and wall sits.

This program is life changing. I took on this challenge knowing that I had some limitations that I needed to overcome, and I was able to accomplish my goals in a short period of time. This has never happened before. The amount of weight that I lost is incomprehensible. My confidence has been restored and for that, I am very grateful.

I would tell people considering this program to challenge yourself to accomplish what you think is impossible, and never ever give up on yourself or the goals that you set. Nothing worth having comes easy. It takes a made-up mind, faith, and tenacity to prevail. More important, believe that you will achieve...your life has purpose, so strive to be the best you.

> This program is life changing. The amount of weight that I lost is incomprehensible. Challenge yourself to accomplish what you think is impossible, and never ever give up on yourself or the goals that you set.

BICYCLE

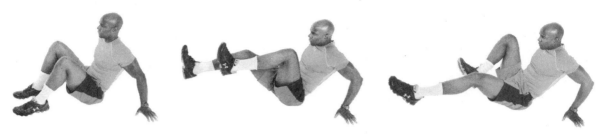

This exercise targets the upper and lower abs, including obliques.

Sit with your knees bent and hands next to your body, palms down. Lift your feet off the floor so that your shins are parallel to the ground and your knees make 90-degree angles. Breathe normally and bring your left knee toward your chest as you extend your right leg all the way; then bring your right knee toward your chest as you extend your left leg.

Perform the move smoothly for 20 to 40 seconds for 3 to 4 sets.

SCISSOR

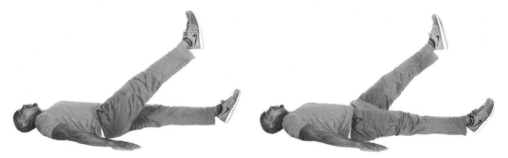

This exercise targets the upper and lower abs.

Lie on your back with your arms next to your hips, palms down. Keeping your core engaged and legs straight, lift both legs off the ground and move your right leg up toward the ceiling while keeping your left leg several inches off the ground. Breathe normally as you lower your right leg toward the ground, then lift your left leg toward the ceiling (like a pair of scissors opening and closing) while keeping your right leg several inches off the ground. Keep your back pressed against the floor to protect your lower back.

Perform smoothly for 20 to 40 seconds for 3 to 4 sets.

CRUNCH

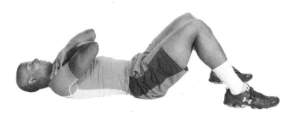

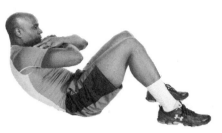

This exercise targets the upper and lower abs.

Lie on your back, knees bent, and cross your arms over your chest. Slowly lift your shoulders off the ground high enough so that your shoulder blades clear the ground; pause for 1 second, then lower your upper body back down.

Do 20 to 30 reps for 3 to 4 sets.

From Morris:

Everybody wants the abs, but nobody wants to do what they need to get them! Guys will be in the gym all day long and hit the weights and max out on their bench, but that's not gonna do it. It's all about the diet if you want those abs.

IN AND OUT

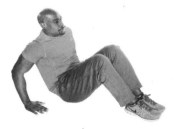

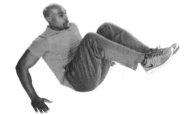

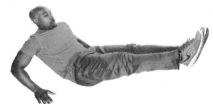

This exercise targets the upper and lower abs, including obliques.

Sit on the floor with your hands on the floor near your hips and your legs extended in front of you. Bend your knees and draw your knees up toward your chest; pause briefly and then lower your legs to the floor, maintaining the bend in your knees.

Perform the move for 20 to 40 seconds for 3 to 4 sets.

From Obi:

There is no such thing as spot reduction, meaning you can't remove belly fat by doing ab exercises! These exercises will make your abs stronger, but you have to lower your overall body fat through diet and exercise to eliminate the fat around your midsection—or anywhere else on your body.

SIT-UP

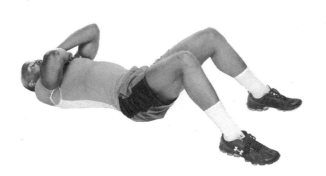 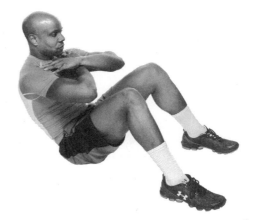

This exercise targets the upper and lower abs.

Lie on your back with your knees bent and your hands interlaced behind your head or arms crossed over your chest. (You can place your feet under a couch or piece of furniture for stability if you like.) Exhale as you slowly bring your torso off the ground to bring your chest to your knees; lower yourself to the ground as you inhale.

Perform this move for 20 to 30 seconds; that's 1 set. Do 3 to 4 sets.

GYM AB EXERCISES

KNEELING CABLE CRUNCH
(uses cable machine)

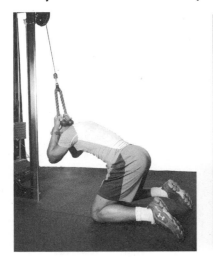 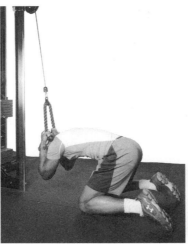 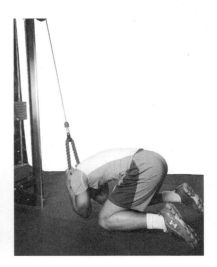

This exercise targets the upper and lower abs.

Connect a rope attachment to a high pulley cable. Kneel on the ground and hinge forward from the hips so your torso is parallel to the ground, holding the rope with both hands next to your ears with your arms bent. Exhale as you slowly contract your abs and pull downward on the cable to bring your elbows to your knees; inhale as you return to the starting position.

Do 15 to 20 reps for 3 to 4 sets.

LEG RAISE
(uses Roman chair)

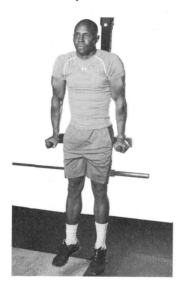 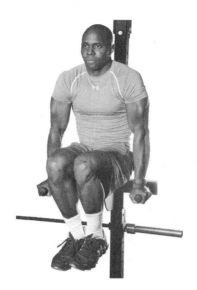

This exercise targets the upper and lower abs and hip flexors.

Place your back against the pad and step up so that your body weight is supported on your forearms. Bend your knees to lift your feet up toward the ceiling until you make 90-degree angles with your hips. Then lower them, pause, and repeat.

Do 12 to 20 reps for 3 to 4 sets.

Part Four

Think to Get Cut

What happens after the first 12 weeks of The Cut? Not only have you changed your body from the inside out, and shed excess body fat while building a sexy, sculpted physique, you've created new, healthy habits. You know how to eat (and how not to eat!) and you know how to exercise. It's those habits and your positive, confident mind-set that will carry you into the coming months, even years.

The last section of the book teaches you how to stay lean—forever! The final two chapters of the book are chapter 15, frequently asked questions about The Cut, and chapter 16, about how to embrace the Cut mind-set for life!

15 Frequently Asked Questions

You've been given the diet and exercise components of the program. You know that if you follow both components, you will lose weight—a phenomenal amount of weight—in the next 12 weeks. Let's address some commonly asked questions we hear about the Cut program:

Q: You mentioned that on the beginner exercise program, you won't burn as many calories as on the intermediate or advanced program. Can I still lose weight on the beginner exercise program?

A: Certainly. The diet you follow is based on your starting weight, and will ensure that you lose weight on The Cut. Because you're exercising only three times a week—not four or five times a week—though, you won't burn as many calories through exercise as people who are working out more. Anyone who follows The Cut needs to stick to the diet plan, but it's especially critical for beginners who want optimal results.

Q: Can I drink coffee before I do my cardio?

A: While research suggests that caffeine before exercise can improve the quality of your workout, it's better to have coffee before you lift weights, not before cardio. The reason? Caffeine can contribute to dehydration, and people sweat more doing cardio than lifting weights. If you like to drink coffee before working out, make sure you drink plenty of water to maintain hydration and prevent muscle cramps.

Q: How much weight can I expect to lose on The Cut?

A: Follow the plan to the letter and you will likely lose a minimum of 1 to 2 pounds per week. Most people who do The Cut lose much more than that, especially during the first four weeks on the program. Your weight loss average may drop after the first 4 weeks or so, but you should continue to lose weight steadily for the entire 12 weeks!

Q: I'm in my 60s. Can I do The Cut?

A: Yes! Any person of any age can follow this program; that's why we have programs for beginner, intermediate, and advanced levels. If you haven't exercised in years, though, or if you're over the age of 40, it's smart to get your doctor's okay before you start exercising. The same goes if you have a medical condition that may affect your ability to work out.

Q: You're both guys. Is this program really for both men and women?

A: Of course! We wanted to create a program that both sexes could do. If you're part of a couple and you both want to get in shape, why not do it together? Remember that men will lose body fat and build lean muscle and women will lose body fat and develop toned, lean bodies as a result of this program. Working out together and eating healthy meals together is a great way to strengthen your bond as you get healthier.

Q: How long will it take me to see results on The Cut?

A: You should see results on the scale in the first week; in fact, your biggest weight loss will probably occur in the first four weeks on the program. You should also see a difference in energy level and overall mood within a week or so.

Q: My time to work out in the morning is limited. Can I break up the workout into two parts?

A: Yes, if that works better for your schedule. Do the strength-training component of the program first to produce the most EPOC response and to save your energy for the rest of your day. It's easier to do cardio at the end of the day, as it takes less mental focus. If you do split up the workouts, drink your protein shake after your strength-training workout.

Q: I notice we're supposed to take fish oil every morning with breakfast. What's the deal with that?

A: Fish oil contains omega-3 fatty acids, which are essential for good health. Most people don't consume enough omega-3 fats, so we include them on The Cut to help reduce your risk of heart disease, stroke, and other health conditions. These fats also help lubricate your joints, which makes them a smart supplement for when you're exercising regularly.

Q: I'm never hungry in the morning. Do I *have* to eat breakfast?

A: Yup. Eating breakfast gives you energy for the morning. If you don't want to eat when you first wake up, that's fine—but make it your goal to eat a morning meal within two hours of waking.

Q: The diet looks great, but I'm not a big exercise person. You said diet is more important than exercise for weight loss, so can't I skip the workout part of the program and just diet instead?

A: Not if you want optimal results! Diet and exercise are both equally important for your overall weight loss. Exercising throughout the 12 weeks does several important things. First, it burns calories and gets you in the habit (a very healthy habit!) of making workouts part of your weekly routine. Even more important, the workouts you do will help you build and retain the lean muscle that is metabolically active—and that means you won't hit a weight loss plateau. The Cut is based on the research that proves that for maximum weight loss, you want to combine a healthy, calorically reduced diet and exercise. The formula is simple:

Healthy, lower-calorie diet + cardio exercise + weight training = maximum weight loss!

From Morris:

As human beings navigating through life, we all have our ups and downs. Working in Hollywood, I get rejected and criticized more often than you'd think. I have bad auditions or bad reviews. When that happens, I tell myself that it's okay to have a pity party—but my pity party doesn't last long.

I'll be honest: There are times when I eat emotionally or reach for junk food out of stress or as a result of a bad day. Sometimes it even happens when we're on set and a scene didn't come out the way I wanted. In those moments of vulnerability, yeah, I'll have some sweets. Or I scarf down some McDonald's. Sometimes I just need that treat! But then I move on and get back to business. If you want to be successful, you have to do the same thing.

Q: I blew it! I'm five weeks into the program and went off the diet for several days. I feel like I've ruined all my hard work. What should I do?

A: Don't worry about it—this happens sometimes! A couple of days being off the diet will not destroy your five weeks of hard work. You just have to make sure that this doesn't become a habit and doesn't derail your progress and motivation. You can still be successful on this program even with a couple of off days, so long as you get back on track with the diet and exercise plan!

Q: My son is 16 years old and wants to lose weight. Can he follow The Cut?

A: Yes, but we would be careful in putting a 16-year-old growing boy on a low-calorie diet. Kids and teens need as many nutrients as possible; talk to your son's doctor about the appropriate calories he should consume each day if he wants to lose weight.

Q: I'm a vegetarian. Can I do The Cut?

A: Of course. You'll just have to use vegetarian options for protein instead of things like chicken, turkey, steak, and fish. Tofu, nonfat Greek yogurt, and low-fat cottage cheese are all good vegetarian protein options.

Q: I couldn't finish the first couple of workouts. What should I do?

A: Listen to your body; do as much as you can, but stop when you're extremely uncomfortable, feel like you can't continue, or start to have pain. You don't have to kill yourself to get in good shape on The Cut! Everyone who does the program has a different level of fitness, so focus on what you're able to do and try to continually improve; within a few weeks, you should notice a significant increase in your strength and cardio fitness level.

Q: I was so sore after my first workout! What's the deal?

A: When you first do a challenging workout that you've never done before, it's normal to have some soreness the first couple of days. As your body gets used to training, you should notice less soreness.

Q: Can I use alcohol as one of my cheat meals?

A: We're okay with a glass of red wine as part of your cheat meal, but suggest that you avoid beer and mixed drinks. The latter are high in calories, and drinking alcohol may encourage you to overdo it with your cheat meal or to abandon your healthy diet altogether!

Q: **I overdid it during one of my workouts and strained my shoulder. What should I do?**

A: Take a couple of days of rest from working out if you believe you strained your shoulder or have any other injury. If it's continuing to bother you five to seven days later, have your doctor check it out.

16 Making the Cut for Life

Congratulations! You made it. And you may be surprised at how quickly the 12 weeks went by.

As you saw from the "Making the Cut" transformation stories, and may have experienced firsthand, the first few weeks of The Cut are the most challenging. Changing your eating habits and getting into a workout groove take mental focus and discipline. Once you pushed through those initial few weeks, though, you found that it got easier—because you created new habits for yourself.

From Morris:

In my mind, I always feel like I have an edge in business and other things I do because I have a strong work ethic. The other day, I had a really long day on set. The next morning, I woke up at four o'clock and I did not want to go to the gym. I didn't have any energy. Well, I got up and I got my butt to the gym. Even if I just ride the bike lightly for 30 minutes, I'm there. That kind of hard work is my edge.

Your mission now? To stick to those healthy habits, as best you can. Eating right and exercising regularly should be a part of your day-to-day life, just like taking a shower or brushing your teeth.

But we know that life happens. We recognize there will be times when you slip up and eat stuff you know isn't great for you. Maybe work responsibilities or family commitments get in the way of your regular workout routine or you went a little crazy on vacation. Stuff happens. When it does, don't beat yourself up. Look at what you can do to get back on track. Maybe it's making time to get to the gym. Maybe it's a week or two of eating clean to get your weight back down. If you need a full-blown jump start, you can always start the program again. It's here for you, whenever you need it.

Making the Cut: Real People, Real Results

Name: William Scott Carter
Age: 42
Location: San Antonio, Texas
Occupation: Self-employed/AdvoCare and front desk at a local gym
Height: 5'10"
Starting weight: 250 pounds
Ending weight: 216.8 pounds

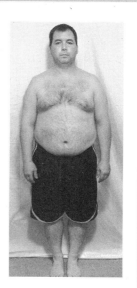

I've been overweight for about 15 years. I've tried dieting without exercise; I've tried diets where you had to purchase special foot to eat; and I did a 12-week program that I did well with but I had to get through it twice to get the results I wanted. I ended up gaining the weight back.

I was really excited about The Cut because I know Obi is the real deal—a true expert who knows what he's talking about. I had been following him on social media for a while and was familiar with him and his work. Since I've had some experience working out in the past, I was really looking forward to getting back into the gym.

Eating healthy on The Cut wasn't really an issue for me.

I made sure I always had healthy food available by keeping easy, ready-to-go items stocked. For example, I always kept celery and peanut butter for snacks when I needed something right away as well as apples and bananas. I had individual packets of meal replacement shakes available in case I didn't have time to heat up a lunch. I also cooked all

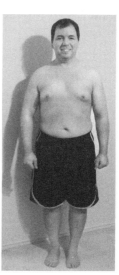

my food on Sunday, saved it in containers, and placed it in the fridge, ready to go. My lunches were mostly prepped into containers for the week.

Getting a workout in after really long days was challenging at times. At the end of a long day—and there were many of those—there is nothing that sounds better than to lie down and sleep. But I had several motivating factors. One, I had to prove to myself and my family that I could actually pull this off. Until now, I've never been able to finish a 12-week program with significant results (and I've tried several over the years). Honestly, I've never really completed anything. I wanted to show my children that anything is possible if you give it everything you have and you don't give up.

Second, I made my goals public, and there were a lot of my family and friends watching my progress. I couldn't allow myself to fail. That alone got me out of the house and to the gym on those nights when I just wanted to sleep. Third, I wanted to be an example of what is possible if you work hard, don't give up, and honestly give it everything you've got. It wasn't easy and there were a couple of times when I did just sleep it off. But when I woke up the next morning, I felt so guilty about missing my workout. I cheated on myself and I hated that feeling.

One thing is certain—for every workout session I pulled off at the end of a long day when I didn't feel like doing it, I felt so good afterward and I was always glad I went. It was the greatest feeling!

At the beginning of the program, I was so out of shape, I couldn't even finish some of the workout routines. I couldn't complete the ab work at all and I think I got about 20 minutes into my cardio before I was exhausted. My body was completely spent. Now that the program is over, I feel like I can't get enough! An hour of cardio is easy...my strength has increased and just this morning I did 100 crunches and 100 scissor kicks without rest!

After 12 weeks, I feel amazing! I can run up several flights of stairs without getting winded when before I would be out of breath just walking up a set of stairs. My body has shrunk significantly and I am much more confident in myself. At 42, I'm very positive about my future and what I will be able to accomplish personally, physically, spiritually, and professionally.

This program basically jump-started an entirely new way of living for me. I was just barely starting to get into the fitness lifestyle. I couldn't stand the work I was doing, so I quit my job and I was in the middle of changing careers when this program came into my life. With the changes I've been able to make, I hope to be able to inspire my friends, family, and anyone else I can...I'm so excited about my future and I truly have a new passion for life!

I can run up several flights of stairs without getting winded when before I would be out of breath just walking up a set of stairs. I am much more confident in myself.

The Cut is 12 weeks for several reasons. One is that this is enough time for you to shed a significant amount of fat and fire up your metabolism with lean muscle so that you're burning more calories every day, all day. Twelve weeks is also long enough for you to develop new healthy habits. Think about it. You no longer have to think about what to have for meals, do you? Your diet has become the norm for you. You look forward to your cheat meals without worrying that you'll blow your diet or ruin your progress. And instead of wondering whether you'll work out—or making excuses as to why you can't—exercise is part of your routine.

STAYING LEAN FOR LIFE

We realize that you're not going to stay on The Cut forever. Once you reach your desired weight, you can maintain it by switching to a maintenance lifestyle program. That means you consume more calories than you did on The Cut while continuing to follow the basic healthy eating principles—basing your diet on lean protein, some healthy fats, and a balance of starchy and fibrous carbs. Yes, you can still have your cheats, as long as you keep those portions small.

Just how much should you eat on maintenance? That will depend on your body weight and your activity level. In general, to maintain your new, leaner body, you should:

- Consume 12 to 14 calories per pound per day if you're exercising twice a week or less;

- Consume 14 to 16 calories per pound per day if you're exercising three or four times a week; and
- Consume 16 to 18 calories per pound per day if you're exercising at least five days a week.

From Obi:

Want to feel and look younger? Exercise is the best "drug" you'll ever take to slow the aging process and keep you feeling, looking, and thinking youthful.

You've learned how to Cut—and now that you know how, you can use these strategies for the rest of your life. So enjoy your new body—and the compliments from people who want to know how you got so fit, so fast. When they ask for *your* secret, tell them about this book!

You can see the results in the mirror, but the real results of The Cut go beyond what you look like. By completing the program, you also now have more energy, more confidence, and overall better health.

From Obi:

I've been very successful in this business, but I don't do it for the money. I love to train people and teach them about healthy diets because it gives me the ability to help improve someone's body, mind, and self-confidence. Anytime you have the ability to make someone healthier on both the inside and the outside, it is a beautiful thing. You can't put a price tag on that!

One of the most rewarding aspects of this program—and why we're so excited about it—is that it changes not only how you look, but how you *feel*. As we said early in the book, this program is simple. That doesn't mean it's easy. Completing the 12-week Cut has proven that you can set challenging goals—and meet them. That's a game changer.

We've seen how people just like you change not only their outward appearances but their inner attitudes as well after doing The Cut. They've learned that they can handle a challenge. That they are stronger than they realized. That they have the ability to overcome obstacles. That gives people an amazing level of self-confidence!

How about you? Now that you've completed The Cut, what's next for you? Maybe it's time to set a new goal for yourself. Maybe that means changing jobs or seeking a promotion. Maybe it means going back to school. Maybe it means setting new goals for your workouts. It might simply mean feeling proud when you look in the mirror—and confident when you take your shirt off!

Whatever your success means to you, embrace it. You worked for it. You earned it. You deserve it. We knew you could do it, and now you know that, too.

So get Cut—and stay Cut—for life!

References

Al-Khudairy, L., L. Hartley, C. Clar, N. Flowers, L. Hooper, and K. Rees. "Omega 6 fatty acids for the primary prevention of cardiovascular disease." *Cochrane Database Systemic Review* 11 (November 16, 2015): CD011094.

Bahr, R. "Excess postexercise oxygen consumption—magnitude, mechanisms and practical implications." *Acta Physiologica Scandinavica. Supplementum* 605 (1992): 1–70.

Barrett, S. J. "The role of omega-3 polyunsaturated fatty acids in cardiovascular health." *Alternative Therapies in Health and Medicine* 19, supplement 1 (2013): 26–30.

Bielinski, R., Y. Schutz, and E. Jéquier. "Energy metabolism during the postexercise recovery in man." *American Journal of Clinical Nutrition* 42, no. 1 (July 1985): 69–82.

Børsheim, E., and R. Bahr. "Effect of exercise intensity, duration and mode on post-exercise oxygen consumption." *Sports Medicine* 33, no. 14 (2003): 1037–60.

Boutcher, S. H. "High-intensity intermittent exercise and fat loss." *Journal of Obesity* (2011): 868305.

Choi, Y., Y. Chang, S. Ryu, J. Cho, S. Rampal, Y. Zhang, J. Ahn, J. A. Lima, H. Shin, and E. Guallar. "Coffee consumption and coronary artery calcium in young and middle-aged asymptomatic adults." *Heart* 101, no. 9 (May 2015): 686–91.

Evans, W. J. "What is sarcopenia?" *Journals of Gerontology. Series A, Biological Sciences and Medical Sciences* 50 (November 1995): 5–8.

Evans, W. J., and W. W. Campbell. "Sarcopenia and age-related changes in body composition and functional capacity." *Journal of Nutrition* 123 (1993): 465–68.

Harper, C. R., and T. A. Jacobson. "The fats of life: The role of omega-3 fatty acids in the prevention of coronary heart disease." *Archives of Internal Medicine* 161, no. 18 (October 8, 2001): 2185–92.

Koloverou, E., D. B. Panagiotakos, C. Pitsavos, C. Chrysohoou, E. N. Georgousopoulou, A. Laskaris, and C. Stefanadis. "The evaluation of inflammatory and oxidative stress biomarkers on coffee–diabetes association: Results from the 10-year follow-up of the ATTICA Study (2002–2012)." *European Journal of Clinical Nutrition* 69 (November 2015): 1220–25.

Laforgia, J., R. T. Withers, and C. J. Gore. "Effects of exercise intensity and duration on the excess post-exercise oxygen consumption." *Journal of Sports Sciences* 24, no. 12 (2006): 1247–64.

Marcell, T. J. "Sarcopenia: Causes, consequences, and preventions." *Journal of Gerontology: Medical Sciences* 58, no. 10 (2003): M911–16.

Minaker, K. L. "Common clinical sequelae of aging." Chapter 24 in L. Goldman and A. I. Schafer, eds. *Goldman's Cecil Medicine*, 24th edition. Philadelphia: Elsevier Saunders, 2011.

Perry, C. G. R., G. J. F. Heigenhauser, A. Bonen, and L. L. Spriet. "High-intensity aerobic interval training increases fat and carbohydrate metabolic capacities in human skeletal muscle." *Applied Physiology, Nutrition, and Metabolism* 33, no. 6 (2008): 1112–23.

Scott, C. B., and R. B. Kemp. "Direct and indirect calorimetry of lactate oxidation: Implications for whole-body energy expenditure." *Journal of Sports Sciences* 23, no. 1 (January 2005): 15–19.

Shah, K., and D. T. Villareal. "Obesity." Chapter 83 in H. M. Fillit and K. Rockwood, eds. *Brocklehurst's Textbook of Geriatric Medicine and Gerontology*, 7th edition. Philadelphia: Elsevier Saunders, 2010.

Tabata, I., K. Nishimura, M. Kouzaki, et al. "Effects of moderate-intensity endurance and high-intensity intermittent training on anaerobic capacity and VO$_2$ max." *Medicine and Science in Sports and Exercise* 28, no. 10 (1996): 1327–30.

Tremblay, A., J.-A. Simoneau, and C. Bouchard. "Impact of exercise intensity on body fatness and skeletal muscle metabolism." *Metabolism* 43, no. 7 (1994): 814–18.

https://nccih.nih.gov/health (accessed December 1, 2015).

Converting to Metrics

Volume Measurement Conversions

Cups	Tablespoons	Teaspoons	Milliliters
		1 tsp	5 ml
1/16 cup	1 tbsp	3 tsp	15 ml
1/8 cup	2 tbsp	6 tsp	30 ml
1/4 cup	4 tbsp	12 tsp	60 ml
1/3 cup	5 1/3 tbsp	16 tsp	75 ml
1/2 cup	8 tbsp	24 tsp	125 ml
2/3 cup	10 2/3 tbsp	32 tsp	155 ml
3/4 cup	12 tbsp	36 tsp	175 ml
1 cup	16 tbsp	48 tsp	250 ml

Weight Measurement Conversions

US	Metric
1 ounce	28.4 grams (g)
8 ounces	227.5 g
16 ounces (1 pound)	455 g

Cooking Temperature Conversions

Celsius/Centigrade	F = (C x 1.8) + 32
Fahrenheit	C = (F−32) x 0.5555

Zero degrees Celsius and 100°C are arbitrarily placed at the melting and boiling points of water, while Fahrenheit establishes 0°F as the stabilized temperature when equal amounts of ice, water, and salt are mixed. So, for example, if you are baking at 350°F and want to know that temperature in Celsius, the following calculation will provide it: C = (350−32) x 0.5555 = 176.66°C.

Index

Page numbers in italics refer to photographs and illustrations in the text.

About the Authors

Morris Chestnut has enjoyed tremendous critical and commercial success as a film and television star for more than two decades. He is best known for his roles in films such as *Boyz n the Hood*, *The Brothers*, *The Perfect Holiday*, *Think Like a Man*, the commercially and critically acclaimed *The Best Man* and its successful sequel, *The Best Man Holiday*, and *The Perfect Guy*. Chestnut stars in the title role in Fox's series *Rosewood* as a Miami pathologist who teams up with the police to solve the city's most challenging cases.

In 2013, he starred opposite Halle Berry in TriStar's *The Call*. That same year, he also starred in Universal's *Kick-Ass 2* opposite Jim Carrey and Chloë Grace Moretz, and the studio's tentpole summer comedy, *Identity Thief*, with Melissa McCarthy. His television credits include TNT's *Legends*, FX's *American Horror Story*, and Showtime's *Nurse Jackie*. His other films include Screen Gems' *When the Bough Breaks* and the thriller *Heist*, directed by Scott Mann.

Obi Obadike is a celebrity fitness and nutrition expert who has graced the cover of over 50 fitness magazines and has authored more than 100 articles for fitness magazines, making him one of the most published fitness experts over the last 10 years. He has trained and dieted some of the most influential celebrities in the world.

He was recognized in January 2016 as the most influential expert in the fitness and health space in the world on Twitter by a top social media analytics site called Onalytica. He was named Writer of the Year for the largest Internet site in the world in Bodybuilding.com in 2012. In January 2014, he was recognized as one of the top 10 most influential fitness experts on the Web by Dr. Oz's Sharecare.com. In April 2016, he, along with Jack LaLanne, Arnold Schwarzenegger, and Jillian Michaels, was named one of the top 10 most inspirational fitness personalities by AskMen.com. Also in 2016, he was selected as one of the top 50 fittest people in the world by AskMen.com.

Obadike was the co-host and judge (with Jillian Michaels and Randy Hetrick, founder and CEO of TRX) on a fitness reality competition show called *Sweat Inc.* that premiered on Spike TV in fall 2015. He is the current co-host of a nationally syndicated Health TV show called *Lifestyle Magazine*, which airs every Thursday on TBN, the Family Channel, Hope Channel, and other nationally syndicated networks. The show is aired in 190 countries.

Obidake was a top Division I collegiate track athlete at Cal State Fullerton, where he was the school record holder in the 100 and 200 meters as well as the 400-meter relay. He was also co-athlete of the year at the university and a two-time All Big West Conference sprinter. He holds BA/BS and MS degrees and is a certified nutritionist specialist and certified trainer with ISSA. He has written for and contributed to fitness magazines and websites, including *Muscle & Fitness*, *Shape*, Bodybuilding.com, AskMen.com, Sharecare.com, LiveStrong, and many others. His monthly Q-and-A fat loss column in *Muscle & Fitness* magazine launched in April 2016.

Want to know how we get Cut—and stay cut? For motivation tips, follow Morris:

On Twitter: @Morris_Chestnut
On Facebook: MorrisChestnut
On Instagram: @morrischestnutofficial

For motivation, fitness, and weight loss tips, follow Obi:

On Twitter: @Obi_Obadike
On the Web: Obiobadike.com
On Facebook: Obi ObadikeFitness and oobadike
On Instagram: @obiobadike